Indigenous Health Equity and Wellness

T0173902

This book focuses on promoting health equity and addressing health disparities among Indigenous peoples of the United States (U.S.) and associated Territories in the Pacific Islands and Caribbean.

It provides an overview of the current state of health equity across social, physical, and mental health domains to provide a preliminary understanding of the state of Indigenous health equity. Part 1 of the book traces the promotive, protective, and risk factors related to Indigenous health equity. Part 2 reports promising pathways to achieving and transcending health equity through the description of interventions that address and promote wellness related to key outcomes.

The chapters in this book were originally published as a special issue of the *Journal of Ethnic & Cultural Diversity in Social Work*.

Catherine E. McKinley is Associate Professor at the Tulane University School of Social Work.

Michael S. Spencer is Presidential Term Professor at the University of Washington School of Social Work.

Karina L. Walters is Professor and Katherine Chambers Hall University Scholar at the University of Washington School of Social Work.

Charles R. Figley is Professor and Paul Henry Kurzweg, MD Chair in Disaster Mental Health at the Tulane University School of Social Work.

Indigenous Health Equity and Wellness

Edited by
**Catherine E. McKinley, Michael S. Spencer,
Karina L. Walters and Charles R. Figley**

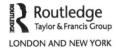

Routledge
Taylor & Francis Group

LONDON AND NEW YORK

First published 2022
by Routledge
4 Park Square, Milton Park, Abingdon, Oxon OX14 4RN

and by Routledge
605 Third Avenue, New York, NY 10158

Routledge is an imprint of the Taylor & Francis Group, an informa business

© 2022 Taylor & Francis

All rights reserved. No part of this book may be reprinted or reproduced or utilised in any form or by any electronic, mechanical, or other means, now known or hereafter invented, including photocopying and recording, or in any information storage or retrieval system, without permission in writing from the publishers.

Trademark notice: Product or corporate names may be trademarks or registered trademarks, and are used only for identification and explanation without intent to infringe.

British Library Cataloguing in Publication Data
A catalogue record for this book is available from the British Library

ISBN: 978-0-367-71483-3 (hbk)
ISBN: 978-0-367-71484-0 (pbk)
ISBN: 978-1-003-15227-9 (ebk)

DOI: 10.4324/9781003152279

Typeset in Minion Pro
by Newgen Publishing UK

Publisher's Note
The publisher accepts responsibility for any inconsistencies that may have arisen during the conversion of this book from journal articles to book chapters, namely the inclusion of journal terminology.

Disclaimer
Every effort has been made to contact copyright holders for their permission to reprint material in this book. The publishers would be grateful to hear from any copyright holder who is not here acknowledged and will undertake to rectify any errors or omissions in future editions of this book.

Contents

Citation Information

The chapters in this book were originally published in the *Journal of Ethnic & Cultural Diversity in Social Work*, volume 30, issue 1–2 (2021). When citing this material, please use the original page numbering for each article, as follows:

For any permission-related enquiries please visit:
www.tandfonline.com/page/help/permissions

Notes on Contributors

Xochilt Alamillo, Graduate School of Social Work, University of Denver, Denver, Colorado, USA.

Antonia R. G. Alvarez, School of Social Work, Portland State University, Portland, OR, USA.

Mike Anastario, Universidad Centroamericana José Simeón Cañas, Antiguo Cuscatlán, La Libertad, El Salvador.

Matilda M. Antone, Department of Social Work, Myron B. Thompson School of Social Work, University of Hawai'i at Mānoa, Honolulu, Hawai'i, USA.

Joyell Arscott, White Clay (A'aninin) Nation, Johns Hopkins University School of Nursing, Baltimore, MD, USA.

Meredith E. Bagwell-Gray, University of Kansas School of Social Welfare, Lawrence, KS, USA.

Ramona E. Beltrán, Graduate School of Social Work, University of Denver, Denver, Colorado, USA.

Kathryn L. Braun, Public Health and Social Work, Office of Public Health Studies and Hā Kūpuna National Resource Center for Native Hawaiian Elders, Thompson School of Social Work & Public Health, University of Hawai'i at Mānoa, Honolulu, HI, USA.

Teresa Brockie, White Clay (A'aninin) Nation, Johns Hopkins University School of Nursing, Baltimore, MD, USA.

Colette V. Browne, Social Work, Department of Social Work and Hā Kūpuna National Resource Center for Native Hawaiian Elders, Thompson School of Social Work & Public Health, University of Hawai'i at Mānoa, Honolulu, HI, USA.

Rachel L. Burrage, Department of Social Work and Hā Kūpuna National Resource Center for Native Hawaiian Elders, Thompson School of Social Work & Public Health, University of Hawai'i at Mānoa, Honolulu, HI, USA.

Jacquelyn Campbell, White Clay (A'aninin) Nation, Johns Hopkins University School of Nursing, Baltimore, MD, USA.

Rachel Clarke, Community-Based Research Institute, Florida International University, Miami, Florida, USA.

Lisa Colón, Graduate School of Social Work, University of Denver, Denver, Colorado, USA.

Genevieve Cox, Department of Health and Human Development, Montana State University, Bozeman, Montana, USA.

Gail Dana-Sacco, Passamaquoddy Tribe, Johns Hopkins University, Center for American Indian Health, Baltimore, MD, USA.

Celina M. Doria, School of Social Service Administration, University of Chicago, Chicago, Illinois, USA.

Tessa Evans-Campbell, School of Social Work, University of Washington, Seattle, Washington, USA.

Angela R. Fernandez, School of Nursing, University of Wisconsin, Madison, WI.

Charles R. Figley, School of Social Work, Tulane University, New Orleans, Louisiana, USA.

Paula Firemoon, Fort Peck Community College, Poplar, Montana, USA.

Nancy Glass, White Clay (A'aninin) Nation, Johns Hopkins University School of Nursing, Baltimore, MD, USA.

Ramey Growing Thunder, Fort Peck Tribes Language and Culture Department, Fort Peck Community College, Poplar, Montana, USA.

Shannon Holder, Department of Health and Human Development, Montana State University, Bozeman, Montana, USA.

Michelle M. Hospital, Community-Based Research Institute, Florida International University, Miami, Florida, USA.

Brittany Wenniserí:iostha Jock, Kanien'kehaka (Mohawk), School of Human Nutrition, Centre for Indigenous Peoples' Nutrition and Environment (CINE), McGill University, Montreal, Quebec, CA.

Olivia Johnson, Fort Peck Community College, Poplar, Montana, USA.

Michelle Johnson-Jennings, College of Arts and Science, University of Saskatchewan, Saskatoon, Canada.

Kristin N. M. Kaniaupio, Department of Social Work, Myron B. Thompson School of Social Work, University of Hawai'i at Mānoa, Honolulu, Hawai'i, USA.

Em Loerzel, White Earth Anishinaabekwe, University of Washington, Seattle, WA, USA.

John Lowe, Indigenous Nursing Research for Health Equity, Florida State University, Tallahassee, Florida, USA.

Catherine E. McKinley, School of Social Work, Tulane University, New Orleans, Louisiana, USA.

Jill Messing, Arizona State University School of Social Work, Phoenix, AZ, USA.

Noreen Mokuau, Hā Kūpuna National Resource Center for Native Hawaiian Elders, Myron B. Thompson School of Social Work & Public Health, University of Hawai'i at Mānoa, Honolulu, HI, USA.

Sandra L. Momper, School of Social Work, University of Michigan, Ann Arbor, Michigan, USA.

Staci L. Morris, Community-Based Research Institute, Florida International University, Miami, Florida, USA.

Shelley Muneoka, Hā Kūpuna National Resource Center for Native Hawaiian Elders, Thompson School of Social Work & Public Health, University of Hawai'i at Mānoa, Honolulu, HI, USA.

Kira L. Rapozo, Department of Social Work, Myron B. Thompson School of Social Work, University of Hawai'i at Mānoa, Honolulu, Hawai'i, USA.

Adriann Ricker, Fort Peck Community College, Poplar, Montana, USA.

Cheryl Riggs, Indigenous Nursing Research for Health Equity, Florida State University, Tallahassee, Florida, USA.

Elizabeth Rink, Department of Health and Human Development, Montana State University, Bozeman, Montana, USA.

Bushra Sabri, White Clay (A'aninin) Nation, Johns Hopkins University School of Nursing, Baltimore, MD, USA.

Jenn Miller Scarnato, School of Social Work, Tulane University, New Orleans, Louisiana, USA.

Katie Schultz, School of Social Work, University of Michigan, Ann Arbor, Michigan, USA.

Michael S. Spencer, School of Social Work University of Washington, Seattle, Washington, USA.

Sandra Stroud, Choctaw Nation Behavioral Health Choctaw Nation of Oklahoma, Talihina, Oklahoma, USA.

Tyran Terada, Hā Kūpuna National Resource Center for Native Hawaiian Elders, Thompson School of Social Work & Public Health, University of Hawai'i at Mānoa, Honolulu, HI, USA.

Michelle G. Thompson, School of Social Policy & Practice, University of Pennsylvania, Philadelphia, Pennsylvania, USA.

Eric F. Wagner, Community-Based Research Institute, Florida International University, Miami, Florida, USA.

Karina L. Walters, School of Social Work University of Washington, Seattle, Washington, USA.

Yan Yan Wu, Office of Public Health Studies and Hā Kūpuna National Resource Center for Native Hawaiian Elders, Thompson School of Social Work & Public Health, University of Hawai'i at Mānoa, Honolulu, HI, USA.

Introduction:

Mental, physical and social dimensions of health equity and wellness among U.S. Indigenous peoples: What is known and next steps

Catherine E. McKinley ⓘD, Michael S. Spencer, Karina L. Walters, and Charles R. Figley

ABSTRACT

This special issue and introduction focuses on promoting health equity and addressing health disparities among Indigenous peoples of the United States (U.S.) and associated Territories in the Pacific Islands and Caribbean. We provide an overview of the current state of health equity across social, physical, and mental health domains. In Part 1 of the special issue, we trace promotive, protective, and risk factors related to Indigenous health equity. Part 2 of the special issue describes interventions that address and promote wellness, providing promising pathways to achieving and transcending health equity.

Health equity is a salient focus within social work research, as evidenced by the American Academy of Social Work & Social Welfare's grand challenge to "Close the Health Gap" (Grand Challenges for Social Work, 2020). In support of this grand challenge and with the collaboration of its co-chairs, Michael Spencer and Karina Walters (Grand Challenges for Social Work, 2020), this special issue focuses on promoting health equity and addressing health disparities among Indigenous peoples of the United States (U.S.) and associated Territories in the Pacific Islands and Caribbean. Specifically, Indigenous peoples of the contiguous U.S. and Alaska (American Indians and Alaska Natives) belong to 574 federally recognized tribes (Bureau of Indian Affairs, 2020), more than 60 state recognized tribes (National Conference on State Legislatures, 2016), and Indigenous groups situated outside either jurisdiction. Moreover, the Indigenous people of Hawai'i (*Kānaka Maoli*) as well as the following Indigenous populations of U.S. associated Pacific Island flagship territories: American Samoa (e.g., *Samoans*) Guam (e.g., *Chamorros*), and the Commonwealth of North Mariana Islands (e.g., Carolinian-*Refaluwasch, Remathau)*, as well as three freely associated states with the U.S.: The Federated States of Micronesia (e.g, *Chuukese, Phnpeian, Kosraean, Yapese*), the Republic of Marshall Islands (e.g., Marshallese- *Aolepān Aorōkin M̧ajeḷ*), and the Republic of Palau (e.g., *Palauans*) constitute at least another 1.4 million Indigenous Peoples. Finally, Indigenous Peoples include the 12, 272 self-identified *Taíno* or "Spanish/Puerto Rican American Indians" of the U.S. Territory of Puerto Rico (U.S. Census, 2010).

American Indian and Alaska Native (AI/AN), Native Hawaiians, and other Indigenous Pacific Island (NHPI) populations are rapidly growing, constituting nearly 2.5% of the total U.S. population (2% AI/AN;.04% NHPI). They are disproportionately young, with about one-third being under the age of 18 in comparison with the one-fourth of the U.S. population overall (US Census, 2012a, 2012b). Although great heterogeneity and resilience exist among AI/AN and NHPI people (hereafter referred to as "Indigenous" when combined), epidemiological data demonstrate these groups suffer devastatingly high rates of health disparities in comparison with other populations. Disparities are linked to land loss, cultural devastations, a lack of access to health environments, insufficient nutrition, and exposure to high levels of environmental contaminants (Walters et al., 2011). AI/ANs are more likely than any other group to die from obesity-related conditions, diabetes, CVD, chronic liver disease, or suicide (Holm et al., 2010). Obesity-related inequity has been linked to alarming disparities in Type 2 Diabetes/T2D and cardiovascular disease among AI/ANs, particularly youth overall (Centers for Disease Control and Prevention, 2014). Moreover, Indigenous populations have the highest rates of smoking and drinking behaviors which are related to a multitude of serious chronic long term health problems. AI/AN youth are particularly vulnerable. They are 1.3 times higher than non-AI/AN peer populations to be obese (Roberts et al., 2009); are much more likely to suffer from serious, lifelong obesity- related illnesses compared to their non-AI/AN peers; and have more than a 70% chance of being obese in adulthood.

In addition, AI/AN youth are much more likely than non-AI/AN youth to initiate alcohol, tobacco, and other drug use (ATOD) at much younger ages and also have higher rates of tobacco use (45% vs 29%) and illicit drug use compared to their non-native peers (Stanley et al., 2014). Additionally, AI/AN youth have the highest suicide rate among all ethnic groups (3x higher) in the U.S., and suicide is the second leading cause of death for AI/AN youth 15–24 years old (Zamora-Kapoor et al., 2016). Overlapping suicide and HIV risk factors, particularly among sexual and gender minority youth, place AI/AN youth at increased risk for suicide and HIV. In fact, HIV diagnosis among gay Indigenous males increased from by 63% from 2005 to 2014 (CDC, 2018). AI/ANs have the shortest time to AIDS diagnosis than any other racial or ethnic group and have the poorest HIV survival rates-reflecting disparities in education, prevention efforts and systems of care. Despite the glaring health disparities, there is a paucity of culturally-grounded research addressing and preventing the health disparities of Indigenous populations. Indigenous populations are dramatically underrepresented in research, particularly in the behavioral science literature, leaving the field with little data on important risk factors, coping behaviors, and health outcomes. Without a larger body of evidence, it will be difficult to identify the strategies and develop the programs necessary to reduce Indigenous health disparities.

Moreover, despite Treaty agreements to provide for the wellness and health of many Indigenous peoples, an absence of clear understanding of the current state of health equity poses a barrier to ameliorating and addressing health disparities. A lack of culturally relevant and evidence-informed solutions to promote wellness and address these health gaps serves to further exacerbate these inequities. In this introduction to the special issue, we first provide a brief overview of some of the key physical and social/behavioral outcomes relevant for adult Indigenous peoples of the U.S. using a culturally relevant framework. In the articles for Part 1 of this special issue, we track culturally relevant promotive, protective, and risk factors relating to health equity as they relate to the focal outcomes of these articles. In Part 2 of the special issue, we provide articles focused on promising intervention strategies to promote wellness among diverse Indigenous peoples. The focus now turns to a culturally relevant framework for wellness.

The framework of historical oppression, resilience, and transcendence (FHORT)

Health equity among Indigenous populations is inseparable from experiences of historical oppression and cultural disruption imposed by colonization, yet also from the concomitant resilience, transcendence, and strengths of Indigenous Peoples. Thus, the culturally-grounded Framework of Historical Oppression, Resilience and Transcendence (FHORT) developed through over a decade of ethnographic work with Indigenous communities informs the approach to this special issue (Burnette & Figley, 2017). Historical oppression expands upon the prominent concept of historical trauma, which focuses on the massive trauma imposed upon Indigenous peoples historically (Brave Heart et al., 2011; Walters et al., 2011). This expansion delineates forms of oppression, recognizing that historical oppression (a) is localized to the distinct contexts and histories of Indigenous peoples colonized throughout history; and (b) explicitly focused on the forms of oppression that are both historical and contemporary in nature (Burnette & Figley, 2017). These contemporary forms of oppression have not subsided or ended; they continue, are perpetuated, and exacerbated by the harm imposed by colonization through the chronic and cumulative risk factors of economic and environmental marginalization, discrimination and racism, health inequities, chronic stress and trauma, and additional factors (Burnette & Figley, 2017). Health inequities and historical oppression, are thus, highly related and inseparable. Notwithstanding experiences of structural and historical oppression, Indigenous peoples strive for resilience, transcendence, and wellness across mental, emotional, physical, social, and spiritual dimensions.

According to the FHORT, the interconnections and balance across eco-systemic risk, promotive and protective factors (i.e. societal, community, cultural, environmental, familial, relational, and individual) interact and contribute to greater or impaired *wellness* across physical, spiritual, social, and mental dimensions. Some even experience transcendence despite being chronically exposed to historical oppression (See Figure 1). These interrelated risk (i.e., those that worsen or contribute to problems), protective (i.e., those that protect against deleterious or enhance wellness), and promotive factors (i.e., strengths and resources, regardless of whether adversity is present) (Masten, 2018) interact across ecological levels to predict key outcomes related to wellness and health (Burnette & Figley, 2017). Transcendence expands upon the experience of recovering or adapting well, to describe people attaining deeper levels of meaning, life satisfaction, posttraumatic growth, and wholeness, than if they had never experienced adversity (Burnette & Figley, 2017). The FHORT is one culturally congruent framework to address health equity among Indigenous people; other promising frameworks, such as the Indigenist Stress-coping model (Walters et al., 2009) and the Native-Reliance theoretical framework (Lowe, 2002; Lowe et al., 2019) are covered in the issues' articles.

The focus now turns to a brief overview of the current state of health equity across social, physical, and mental health domains. Because Indigenous youth outcomes have been introduced and are systematically covered elsewhere (Burnette & Figley, 2016), these sections focus on adults. This overview is by no means exhaustive, but provides a preliminary understanding of the state of Indigenous health equity with which to situate the remainder of the articles. We then summarize

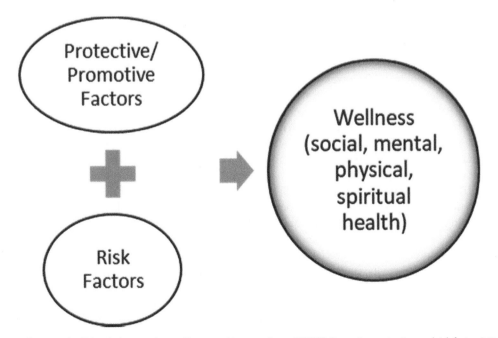

Figure 1. Framework of historical oppression, resilience, and transcendence (FHORT). Promotive, protective, and risk factors interact and occur across ecological (macro [societal, community], meso [familial, agencies], and micro levels [individual]).

the articles contained in Part 1 of the special issue, tracing the promotive, protective, and risk factors related to Indigenous health equity. Finally, we provide an overview of the articles contained in Part 2 of this special issue, reporting promising pathways to achieving and transcending health equity through interventions to address disparities and promote wellness.

Physical wellness promotive, protective, and risk factors

Indigenous health disparities and health risk are in part, due to a complex web of interconnected biological, behavioral, social, and environmental factors acting at multiple levels across the life course. Since the advent of colonization, health equity among Indigenous peoples has been disrupted across social, physical, and mental health dimensions. At present, AIAN[1] death rates are close to 50% greater than for non-Hispanic whites (Centers for Disease Control and Prevention, 2014) and AI/ANs are more likely to experience disabilities than non-Hispanic whites (Siordia et al., 2017). The life-expectancy for AI/ANs hovers around 5.5 years lower than non-AI/ANs (Indian Health Service, 2019). Mortality due to accidents of all types are 2.5 times higher for AI/ANs, and diabetes, alcohol and cirrhosis, and chronic liver related mortality are 3.2, 6.6, and 4.6 times higher than the rate of non-AI/ANs (Indian Health Service, 2019). Several physical contributors to the morbidity and mortality of AI/ANs include obesity, cardiovascular disease (CVD), and associated chronic health conditions related to diabetes, cancer, and stroke (Espey et al., 2014). In this section, we focus on the primary causes of death for AI/ANs including CVD, diabetes, and cancer.

Research documents higher CVD (and the associated risks of physical inactivity, smoking, obesity, hypertension, and cholesterol) for AI/ANs than non-AI/ANs (Center for American Indian Health Research, 2017). Unlike the general U.S. population, CVD has been increasing and is often fatal for AI/ANs, which may be associated with high levels of diabetes among AI/AN peoples (Howard et al., 1999). The Strong Heart Study AI/AN data for 1989 (Welty et al., 2002), 1995, and 2006 reported increasing prevalence for diabetes and hypertension; yet, the intake of fruits or vegetables, smoking rates, and physical inactivity have not significantly changed among AI/AN peoples (Jernigan et al., 2010). Health benefits of eating traditional AI/AN foods versus Western diets indicate culturally-specific factors being relevant (Bersamin et al., 2008).

A recent systematic review also revealed important psychosocial factors related to CVD and associated disorders, such as diabetes (Burnette et al., 2020). Depression, post-traumatic stress disorder (PTSD), anxiety, alcohol and other drug (AOD) abuse were clear risks for CVD, obesity, diabetes, and smoking. Moreover, enculturation, social support, and social infrastructures for health were clear protective factors for these outcomes, whereas trauma, such as intimate partner violence (IPV) differentially affected women and men (Burnette et al., 2020). Importantly, enculturation (engagement and identifying with Indigenous culture) tended to be associated with higher levels of physical activity, along with lower levels of hypertension, AOD abuse, stress, and mental distress; in contrast, identifying with mainstream culture was associated with AOD abuse.

The IPV trauma was associated with PTSD, which has been found to contribute to depression and CVD; trauma was also a risk factor for diabetes-management (Burnette et al., 2020). Stress, including experiencing racism and discrimination was a risk factor for obesity, CVD, and diabetes (Burnette et al., 2020). Lower resilience tended to contribute to poorer self-reported health, chronic pain, and depressive symptoms, whereas social support from family and friends tended to be protective, promoting physical activity, and this was especially true for women and children (Burnette et al., 2020). Community infrastructure promoting physical activity promoted exercise, whereas neighborhood poverty tended to contribute to obesity, CVD, and Type 2 diabetes (Burnette et al., 2020). Unsafe communities seem to pose particular threats for women's safety, making public safety in AI/AN communities potentially gendered.

Cancer prevalence and mortality rates differ by gender, region, and tribe (Espey et al., 2014; Plescia et al., 2014). As an example, the incidence of lung cancer continues to increase among AI/AN women despite it decreasing among AI/AN males (Plescia et al., 2014). AI/AN women experience cervical cancer at higher rates, with lower survival rates in comparison with whites (Espey et al., 2005). Further, AI/AN women have not benefited from the same decline in breast cancer death rates that white women have (White et al., 2014). AI/AN men and women both experience elevated incidence of kidney and colorectal cancers, with AI/AN women experiencing higher rates than both white women and AI/AN men (Perdue et al., 2014). Despite colorectal cancer being preventable and treatable, AI/ANs experience the lowest screening rates (Johnson-Jennings et al., 2014). Barriers to cancer screening can include limited private health insurance, low income, and transportation (Espey et al., 2014; Kolahdooz et al., 2014). Though variable, physical health disparities related to CVD, diabetes, cancer, and diabetes tend to be prevalent among many AI/AN peoples, demonstrating the need for culturally and gender-specific ways of addressing such inequities.

Social and mental wellness promotive, protective, and risk factors

AI/ANs also tend to experience elevated social and mental/behavioral health inequities. Along with experiencing elevated risk for severe mental distress, the risk for posttraumatic stress disorder (PTSD) has been found to be two-fold (American Psychological Association, 2010). Suicides, drug-related, and homicide-related deaths all hover around twice that of non-AI/ANs (Indian Health Service, 2019). AI/AN peoples experience a high risk for violence as well with IPV rates being 1.7 times higher than for non-AI/AN women (Breiding et al., 2014). The reported rate for AI/AN child maltreatment is also 1.5 times that of whites (US Department of Health and Human Services, 2013). The National Crime Information Center reports that, in 2016, there were 5,712 reports of missing AI/AN women and girls, yet only 116 cases of these thousands were logged into the U.S. Department of Justice's federal missing persons database (Urban Indian Health Institute, 2018). Murder is the third-leading cause of death among AI/AN women and rates of violence on reservations can be up to ten times higher than the national average (Urban Indian Health Institute, 2018).

PTSD, depression, suicide, and AOD abuse have been found to be elevated for Indigenous peoples of the U.S. (AI/ANs and Native Hawaiians) (Ka'apu & Burnette, 2018). A recent systematic review reported a higher prevalence of PTSD for Indigenous peoples, which likely has to do with greater exposure to trauma as a result of historical oppression creating adverse social environments (Ka'apu & Burnette, 2018). Some studies report PTSD rates at 2–3 times that of non-AI/ANs (Gone & Trimble, 2012) ranging from 15.9%-21.9% due to elevated rates of trauma exposure (Beals et al., 2013; Robin et al., 1997). The rate of PTSD for Native Hawaiians was reported as high as 38% (Norris & Slone, 2007). The risk for PTSD among AI/AN women tends to be twice that of AI/AN men (likely due to IPV) (Ka'apu & Burnette, 2018).

Rates of depression among AI/AN are elevated, ranging from 10%-30% (Evans-Campbell et al., 2012) and among Native Hawaiians, ranging from 8%-12.2% (Salvail & Smith, 2007). Berman (2014) relates that historical oppression is an underlying mechanism driving depressive systems, causing cultural disruptions in the forms of " . . . critical cultural, political, and economic transitions for Alaska Natives (p. S329)." Indeed, other research has found that depressive symptoms are associated with historical loss (Whitbeck et al., 2009) and historical oppression (Burnette et al., 2019). Research reports deaths from suicide being eight-fold higher among AI/ANs than non-AI/ANs (Wexler et al., 2012) and the eighth leading cause of AI/AN mortality (Berman, 2014; O'Keefe et al., 2012; Wexler et al., 2012).

AOD abuse and dependence is reported to be elevated for AI/ANs compared to the general U.S. population (Radin et al., 2015). Radin (2015) reports that historical oppression contributes to the loss of community connectedness, making the revitalization of community and culture to offset this loss essential (Radin et al., 2015). The Centers for Disease Control reports that 'the opioid epidemic' disproportionately impacts AI/ANs (Tipps et al., 2018). Along with trauma exposure, AOD use is a primary contributor to other mental health problems, including depression, anxiety, and PTSD among AI/ANs (Ka'apu & Burnette, 2018). AOD disorders have been found to be associated with increased odds (by two-fold) of depressive and anxiety disorders among AI/ANs (Rieckmann et al., 2012).

In closing, given a context of elevated exposure to trauma and historical oppression, PTSD, depression, suicide, and AOD disorders tend to be more prevalent among AI/ANs than non-AI /ANs (Ka'apu & Burnette, 2018). Culturally relevant protective factors that offset disparities included traditional upbringings and maintaining culture, as well as family and social support (Ka'apu & Burnette, 2018). Considerable overlap exists across risk factors for health outcomes. Trauma, both in the forms of historical oppression and contemporary trauma, is a recurring risk factor across mental, social, and physical health inequities. Risk factors arose across eco-systemic levels, such as: historical oppression and loss, economic and high risk community environments, family challenges, and AOD abuse (Ka'apu & Burnette, 2018). Protective factors tended to focus on cultural, community, and family characteristics. Holistic programs that encompass these tenets are among the most promising interventions.

Interventions to promote health equity

Empirically-informed interventions and health promoting programs to increase health equity for Indigenous peoples are relatively scarce, and those that are culturally relevant are even more limited (Liddell & Burnette, 2017). If Indigenous peoples receive inadequate or culturally incongruent interventions, progress toward health equity may be undermined with harmful or ineffective interventions (Dixon et al., 2007). Despite a need for culturally relevant solutions to the aforementioned disparities, access to programs is limited (Gone & Trimble, 2012).

Historically, programs for Indigenous peoples have been imposed from a non-Indigenous perspective (Burnette & Figley, 2016; Gone & Trimble, 2012; Urban Indian Health Institute, 2014), despite culturally-specific interventions being up to four times more effective than non-targeted interventions (Griner & Smith, 2006). Existing interventions have tended to focus on problems, ignoring the profound strengths and resilience of Indigenous peoples (Yuan et al., 2015). Some Western interventions have relied solely on empirical evidence, negating Indigenous holistic knowledge, which has included teachings of ancestors, spiritual practices, and the cross-generational transmission of coping strategies (Liddell & Burnette, 2017). However, Indigenous communities have demanded development of culturally-based Indigenous health prevention and promotion programs in which Indigenous cultural epistemologies, Knowledges, and practices are "front and center" (K.L. Walters et al., 2020) K. L. Walters et al. (2020) outline how Indigenist worldviews and protocols have already been integrated into Indigenous health interventions by incorporating: (1) Original instructions/ancient teachings; (2) Relational restorative practices; (3) Narrative-embodied transformative processes; and (4) Indigenist community-based participatory research.

Amplifying and building upon Indigenous knowledges has been particularly critical to addressing environmentally based health disparities in Indigenous communities. In fact, the Intergovernmental Panel on Climate Change, the World Health Organization, and the National Congress of American Indians have all sounded the alarm that the Indigenous Peoples of North America and the Pacific Islands will disproportionately bear the impact of severe climate change events (Cordalis & Saugee, 2008; Gamble et al., 2016; Maldonado, 2014). Nearly all Indigenous populations live in areas prone to extreme weather events and have economies, cultural practices, and/or subsistence lifeways that are integrally tied to environments in climate sensitive regions (Crimmins et al., 2016).

Because Indigenous Peoples have sacred, cultural, and subsistence connections to these territories, any environmental losses threaten cultural survival and corresponding physical, mental, cultural, and spiritual health. The confluence of poor environmental, socioeconomic inequities, chronic disease conditions, and imminent threat of climate-related hazards has potentially perilous long-term health consequences. As a result, recognizing the potential protective role of engaging in outdoor-based physical activities and the nutritious diets of our ancestors- through harvesting and preparing traditional "First Foods" and engaging in traditional nature-based outdoor physical activities (e.g., gathering wild edible foods, walking historical trails) have recently become integral components for land-based healing approaches for eradicating health conditions (e.g., diabetes, obesity) driving Indigenous health disparities .

Many Indigenous communities are developing culturally based outdoor activities to stimulate healthful, culturally based activities and increase motivation for healthful living based on ancestral lifeways while also ensuring transmission of traditional ecological knowledge and lifeways to the next generation (K.L. Walters et al., 2020). There is a strong scientific premise for designing health promotion interventions within nature-based environments to enact positive impact on activity levels, self-esteem, and emotional well-being (Barton & Rogerson, 2017). Place-based interventions rooted in experiential learning-in-the-environment are compatible with Indigenous epistemologies and may enhance health prevention efforts and health outcomes as well as reinforce communal sustainable practices. We now provide a brief overview of the contents of Part 1 and Part 2 of this double special issue.

Part 1: promotive, protective, and risk factors for Indigenous health equity

Part 1 investigates culturally relevant risk and protective factors for various Indigenous groups, including AI/AN, NHPI, and Mexican American Indian communities related to alcohol and other drug use, diabetes, HIV, migration, suicide, and wellness. First, in, "A Culturally Informed Scoping Review of Native Hawaiian Mental Health and Emotional Wellbeing Literature," the authors use a culturally-informed approach for their scoping review. The authors' highlight culturally-relevant protective and promotive factors, such as family support, spirituality, culturally-grounded interventions, and connection to place as factors related to psychological wellness. Second, in "What's Love Got to Do with It? "Love" and Alcohol Use among U.S. Indigenous Peoples: Aligning Research with Real-World Experiences," the authors present a mixed-methods examination of Indigenous peoples' experiences of love across two tribes, with love being characterized as a focal component of family resilience. Components of love described in the qualitative research include physical affection, verbal affection, rituals relating to expressing love, and generational changes in love expression. In the quantitative component of the study, love is investigated in the context of an Indigenous-based family resilience framework to understand – commensurate with qualitative results – whether generational changes in such resilience are present and how love is associated with alcohol use.

Third, in "Diabetes, Mental Health, and Utilization of Mental Health Professionals Among Native Hawaiian and Pacific Islander Adults", the authors fill and important gap to evaluate whether diabetes or borderline/prediabetes is associated with serious psychological distress, and whether mental health professional utilization has an interacting effect on this association. Diabetes was associated with positive scoring for serious psychological distress conditioned upon age, sex, partnership status, and educational levels. Mental health stigma, use of non-culturally relevant measures, and exclusion of informal mental support variables may influence precise measurement of mental health symptomatology, creating a need for culturally grounded measurement development among Native Hawaiian and Pacific Islanders.

Fourth, the authors of "Salud, Cultura, Tradicion: Findings from an Alcohol and Other Drug and HIV Needs Assessment in Urban "Mexican American Indian" Communities" describe Mexican American Indian communities and present findings from a needs assessment related to knowledge, stigma, and risk related to these concerns. The important protective functions of cultural identity, healing, and community support are highlighted. Finally, in "Migration and Resilience in Native Hawaiian Elders," the authors investigate how historical oppression has placed many Indigenous peoples in a precarious economic and environmental situation, leading some elders to migrate to the mainland. Reasons for migrating and resilience, with particular emphasis on the protective aspects of family, culture, and financial well-being are the focal cultural strengths identified.

Part 2: promising interventions for Indigenous health equity

In "Togetherness:" The Role of Intergenerational and Cultural Engagement in Urban American Indian and Alaska Native Youth Suicide Prevention," the authors conducted talking circles with AI/AN elders, adults, and youth in an urban environment to uncover suicide prevention strategies and perceptions of suicide within their communities. Themes of the normalization of suicide, the presence of stigma, and the influence of historical oppression and trauma emerged from the talking circles as barriers or risk factors for suicide prevention. The need for cross-generational engagement, and enculturation, including cultural connectedness, are emphasized as promising prevention strategies. The relationship to place as it relates to wellness and health is examined in, "Being on the Walk Put it Somewhere in My Body:" The Meaning of Place in Health for Indigenous Women." Using the Indigenist stress-coping model, which proposes that cultural and spiritual protective factors buffer against stress and poor health outcomes, this article gleans results from an experiential, place-based intervention to understand how participants responded and were affected by being at sites of historical trauma and oppression. In response to this innovative and culturally-grounded experiential intervention, participants reported embodying resilience and connectedness to place as forms of collective resistance and transcendence.

Next, in "The Development and Testing of a Multi-Level, Multi-Component Pilot Intervention to Reduce Sexual and Reproductive Health Disparities in a Tribal Community," an ecological intervention for American Indian youth in the Northwest is presented. Using community-based participatory research (CBPR) with an ecological systems theory framework, this school-based intervention for youth and parents included a cultural mentoring program. A mixed-methods pre-posttest analysis identified positive preliminary data regarding this intervention, namely an increase in parent-child communication surrounding sexual and reproductive health. This work also reports an increase in youth self-efficacy, condom use, and constructive attitudes toward pregnancy. Increasing parent-child communication and the inclusion of elders in such interventions are recommended to enhance youth sexual and reproductive health and wellness.

"SACRED Connections: A University-Tribal Clinical Research Partnership for School-Based Screening and Brief Intervention for Substance Use Problems among Native American Youth," focuses on health inequities related to AOD use among Native American youth. A university-tribal partnership using the Native-Reliance theoretical framework and CBPR, this randomized control trial focused on the intervention's dissemination and implementation. Findings indicate protective results of the Native-Reliance framework in rates of youth alcohol and marijuana use in comparison with the control group. This study indicates promising results of using a culturally adapted motivational interviewing brief intervention for health equity.

Finally, "From myPlan to ourCircle: Adapting a Web-Based Safety Planning Intervention for Native American Women Exposed to Intimate Partner Violence" describe the cultural adaptation of a safety planning intervention for Native American women. The article traces the practices of Indigenous peoples across the nation in its qualitative inquiries to identify culturally-specific risk and protective factors, which then informed a culturally-responsive web-based safety application. The protective factors identified include ethnic identity and culture, social connectedness with other Native women, enculturation, and resilience despite experiencing historical oppression, including historical and contemporary trauma. Risk factors that informed the intervention include a disruption in Native culture and identification, the need to leave family to escape abusive situations, having high thresholds for red flags related to IPV, and the need to balance between the Native and non-Native contexts.

Conclusion

Given the aforementioned health inequities and concomitant risk and protective factors, important implications for programs and policies should be noted. Promotive, protective, and risk factors span across eco-systemic levels, and include structural, historical, and social determinants of health. Programs incorporating protective cultural knowledge may promote wellness in culturally relevant ways. Given the absence of the incorporation of strengths, protective factors, and resilience within a cultural context, a more nuanced approach that considers gender, tribe, and historical oppression is essential. Policies and programs that address the broad socio-structural factors, such as historical oppression (including racism and discrimination) that have given rise to health inequities are imminent. A holistic approach to wellness that includes environmental, psychological, social, physical and spiritual dimensions is promising. Policies and programs that redress historical oppression (including trauma), revitalize environmental and economic growth, and incorporate cultural enrichment and family supports are needed.

Note

1. Much of the research is limited to AI/AN or Native Hawaiians specifically. Thus, when reporting extant research we limit the scope to those peoples reported on in the primary research rather than Indigenous peoples, which would be inclusive of the aforementioned groups.

Acknowledgments

A special thanks to Jessica Liddell and Jenn Miller Scarnato for their important and instrumental contributions to this special issue.

Funding

This work was supported by the Eunice Kennedy Shriver National Institute of Child Health and Human Development [K12HD043451]; National Institute of General Medical Sciences [U54 GM104940].

ORCID

Catherine E. McKinley (iD) http://orcid.org/0000-0002-1770-5088

References

American Psychological Association. (2010). *APA fact sheet, mental health disparities: American Indian and Alaska Natives*. Retrieved from http://www.psych.org/Share/OMNA/Mental-Health-Disparities-Fact-Sheet–American-Indians.aspx

Barton, J., & Rogerson, M. (2017). The importance of greenspace for mental health. *BJPsych International*, 14(4), 79–81. https://doi.org/10.1192/S2056474000002051

Beals, J., Belcourt-Dittloff, A., Garroutte, E. M., Croy, C., Jervis, L. L., Whitesell, N. R., Mitchell, C. M., & Manson, S. M., & AI-SUPERPFP Team. (2013). Trauma and conditional risk of posttraumatic stress disorder in two American Indian reservation communities. *Social Psychiatry and Psychiatric Epidemiology*, 48(6), 895–905. https://doi.org/10.1007/s00127-012-0615-5

Berman, M. (2014). Suicide among young Alaska Native men: Community risk factors and alcohol control. *American Journal of Public Health*, 104(S3), S329–S335. https://doi.org/10.2105/AJPH.2013.301503

Bersamin, A., Luick, B. R., King, I. B., Stern, J. S., & Zidenberg-Cherr, S. (2008). Westernizing diets influence fat intake, red blood cell fatty acid composition, and health in remote Alaskan Native communities in the center for Alaska

Native health study. *Journal of the American Dietetic Association, 108*(2), 266–273. https://doi.org/10.1016/j.jada. 2007.10.046

Brave Heart, M. Y. H., Chase, J., Elkins, J., & Altschul, D. B. (2011). Historical trauma among Indigenous peoples of the Americas: Concepts, research, and clinical considerations. *Journal of Psychoactive Drugs, 43*(4), 282–290. https://doi. org/10.1080/02791072.2011.628913

Breiding, M. J., Chen, J., & Black, M. C. (2014). *Intimate partner violence in the United States—2010*. National Center for Injury Prevention and Control, Centers for Disease Control and Prevention.

Bureau of Indian Affairs. (2020). *About us*. Retrieved from https://www.bia.gov/about-us

Burnette, C. E., & Figley, C. R. (2016). Risk and protective factors related to the wellness of American Indian and Alaska Native youth: A systematic review. *International Public Health Journal, 8*(2), 58–75.

Burnette, C. E., & Figley, C. R. (2017). Historical oppression, resilience, and transcendence: Can a holistic framework help explain violence experienced by Indigenous people? *Social Work, 62*(1), 37–44. https://doi.org/10.1093/sw/ sww065

Burnette, C. E., Ka'apu, K., Miller Scarnato, J., & Liddell, J. (2020). Cardiovascular health among US Indigenous peoples: A holistic and sex-specific systematic review. *Journal of Evidence-based Social Work, 17*(1), 24–48. https://doi.org/10. 1080/26408066.2019.1617817

Burnette, C. E., Renner, L. M., & Figley, C. R. (2019). The framework of historical oppression, resilience and transcendence to understand disparities in depression amongst Indigenous peoples. *The British Journal of Social Work, 49*(4), 943–962. https://doi.org/10.1093/bjsw/bcz041

Center for American Indian Health Research. (2017). *The strong heart study: The largest epidemiologic study of cardiovascular disease in American Indians*. Retrieved from https://strongheartstudy.org/

Centers for Disease Control and Prevention. (2014). *American Indian and Alaska Native death Rates nearly 50 percent greater than those of non-Hispanic whites*. Author. http://Www.Cdc.Gov/Media/Releases/2014/p0422-NatAmerican-Deathrate.Html

Centers for Disease Control and Prevention. (2018). *HIV Surveillance Report, (Preliminary)*, 30. http://www.cdc.gov/hiv/ library/reports/hiv-surveillance.html. Published November 2019. Accessed May 28, 2020.

Cordalis, D., & Saugee, D. B. (2008). The effects of climate change on American Indian and Alaska Native tribes. *Natural Resources and the Environment, 22*(3), 45–49. www.jstor.org/stable/40924927

Crimmins, A. J., Balbus, J. L., Gamble, C. B., Beard, J. E., Bell, J. E., Dodgen, D., et al., (Eds.) (2016). *USGCRP, 2016: The impacts of climate change on human health in the United States: A scientific assessment*. U.S. Global Change Research Program. p. 312. https://doi.org/10.1080/01944363.2016.1218736

Dixon, A. L., Yabiku, S. T., Okamoto, S. K., Tann, S. S., Marsiglia, F. F., Kulis, S., & Burke, A. M. (2007). The efficacy of a multicultural prevention intervention among urban american indian youth in the southwest us. *The Journal of Primary Prevention, 28*(6), 547–568. https://doi.org/10.1007/s10935-007-0114-8

Espey, D. K., Jim, M. A., Cobb, N., Bartholomew, M., Becker, T., Haverkamp, D., & Plescia, M. (2014). Leading causes of death and all-cause mortality in American Indians and Alaska Natives. *American Journal of Public Health, 104*(S3), S303–S311. https://doi.org/10.2105/AJPH.2013.301798

Espey, D. K., Paisano, R., & Cobb, N. (2005). Regional patterns and trends in cancer mortality among American Indians and Alaska Natives, 1990–2001. *Cancer, 103*(5), 1045–1053. https://doi.org/10.1002/cncr.20876

Evans-Campbell, T., Walters, K. L., Pearson, C. R., & Campbell, C. D. (2012). Indian boarding school experience, substance use, and mental health among urban two-spirit American Indian/Alaska Natives. *The American Journal of Drug and Alcohol Abuse, 38*(5), 421–427. https://doi.org/10.3109/00952990.2012.701358

Gamble, J. L., Balbus, J., Berger, M., Bouye, K., Campbell, V., Chief, K., Conlon, K., & Wolkin, A. F. (2016). *Ch.9: Populations of concern. The impacts of climate change on human health in the United States: A scientific assessment*. U.S. Global Change Research Program. pp. 247–286.

Gone, J. P., & Trimble, J. E. (2012). American Indian and Alaska Native mental health: Diverse perspectives on enduring disparities. *Annual Review of Clinical Psychology, 8*(1), 131–160. https://doi.org/10.1146/annurev-clinpsy-032511-143127

Grand Challenges for Social Work. (2020). *Close the health gap*. Retrieved from https://grandchallengesforsocialwork. org/close-the-health-gap/

Griner, D., & Smith, T. B. (2006). Culturally adapted mental health intervention: A meta-analytic review. *Psychotherapy: Theory, Research, Practice, Training, 43*(4), 531. https://doi.org/10.1037/0033-3204.43.4.531

Holm, J. E., Vogeltanz-Holm, N., Poltavski, D., & McDonald, L. (2010). Assessing health status, behavioral risks, and health disparities in Northern Plains American Indians. *Public Health Reports, 125*(1), 68–78. https://doi.org/10.1177/ 003335491012500110

Howard, B. V., Lee, E. T., Cowan, L. D., Devereux, R. B., Galloway, J. M., Go, O. T., Howard, W. J., Rhoades, E. R., Robbins, D. C., Sievers, M. L., & Welty, T. K. (1999). Rising tide of cardiovascular disease in American Indians. *Circulation, 99*(18), 2389–2395. https://doi.org/10.1161/01.CIR.99.18.2389

Indian Health Service. (2019). *Disparities*. Retrieved from https://www.ihs.gov/newsroom/factsheets/disparities/

Jernigan, V. B. B., Duran, B., Ahn, D., & Winkleby, M. (2010). Changing patterns in health behaviors and risk factors related to cardiovascular disease among American Indians and Alaska Natives. *American Journal of Public Health*, *100*(4), 677–683. https://doi.org/10.2105/AJPH.2009.164285

Johnson-Jennings, M. D., Tarraf, W., Xavier Hill, K., & González, H. M. (2014). United States colorectal cancer screening practices among American Indians/Alaska Natives, blacks, and non-Hispanic whites in the new millennium (2001 to 2010). *Cancer*, *120*(20), 3192–3299. https://doi.org/10.1002/cncr.28855

Ka'apu, K. K., & Burnette, C. E. (2018). A systematic review of mental health disparities among adult Indigenous men and women of the U.S.: What is known? *British Journal of Social Work*. 49(4), 880-898. doi:10.1093/bjsw/bcz009

Kolahdooz, F., Jang, S. L., Corriveau, A., Gotay, C., Johnston, N., & Sharma, S. (2014). Knowledge, attitudes, and behaviours towards cancer screening in Indigenous populations: A systematic review. *The Lancet Oncology*, *15*(11), e504–e516. https://doi.org/10.1016/S1470-2045(14)70508-X

Liddell, J., & Burnette, C. E. (2017). Culturally-informed interventions for substance abuse among Indigenous youth in the United States: A review. *Journal of Evidence-Informed Social Work*, 14(5), 329-359. doi: 10.1080/23761407.2017.1335631

Lowe, J. (2002). Cherokee self-reliance. *Journal of Transcultural Nursing*, *13*(4), 287–295. https://doi.org/10.1177/104365902236703

Lowe, J., Wagner, E., Morris, S. L., Thompson, M., Sawant, M., Kelley, M., & Millender, E. (2019). Utility of the Native-Reliance theoretical framework, model, and questionnaire. *Journal of Cultural Diversity*, *26*(2), 61-68.

Maldonado, J. K. (2014). A multiple knowledge approach for adaptation to environmental change: Lessons learned from coastal Louisiana's tribal communities. *Journal of Political Ecology*, *21*(1), 62–81. https://doi.org/10.2458/v21i1.21125

Masten, A. S. (2018). Resilience theory and research on children and families: Past, present, and promise. *Journal of Family Theory & Review*, *10*(1), 12–31. https://doi.org/10.1111/jftr.12255

National Conference on State Legislatures. (2016). *Federal and state recognized tribes*. Retrieved from http://www.ncsl.org/research/state-tribal-institute/list-of-federal-and-state-recognized-tribes.aspx#State

Norris, F. H., & Slone, L. B. (2007). The epidemiology of trauma and PTSD. *Handbook of PTSD: Science and Practice*, 78–98. https://dl.uswr.ac.ir/bitstream/Hannan/130962/1/2007%20-%20Handbook%20of%20PTSD%20-%20Friedman%2C%20Keane%2C%20Resick.pdf#page=94

O'Keefe, V. M., Tucker, R. P., Wingate, L. R., & Rasmussen, K. A. (2012). American Indian hope: A potential protective factor against suicidal ideation. *Journal of Indigenous Research*, *1*(2), 3. https://digitalcommons.usu.edu/kicjir/vol1/iss2/3

Perdue, D. G., Haverkamp, D., Perkins, C., Daley, C. M., & Provost, E. (2014). Geographic variation in colorectal cancer incidence and mortality, age of onset, and stage at diagnosis among American Indian and Alaska Native people, 1990–2009. *American Journal of Public Health*, *104*(S3), S404–S414. https://doi.org/10.2105/AJPH.2013.301654

Plescia, M., Henley, S. J., Pate, A., Underwood, J. M., & Rhodes, K. (2014). Lung cancer deaths among American Indians and Alaska Natives, 1990–2009. *American Journal of Public Health*, *104*(S3), S388–S395. https://doi.org/10.2105/AJPH.2013.301609

Radin, S. M., Kutz, S. H., La Marr, J., Vendiola, D., Vendiola, M., Wilbur, B., Thomas, L. R., & Donovan, D. M. (2015). Community perspectives on drug/alcohol use, concerns, needs, and resources in four Washington state tribal communities. *Journal of Ethnicity in Substance Abuse*, *14*(1), 29–58. https://doi.org/10.1080/15332640.2014.947459

Rieckmann, T., McCarty, D., Kovas, A., Spicer, P., Bray, J., Gilbert, S., & Mercer, J. (2012). American Indians with substance use disorders: Treatment needs and comorbid conditions. *The American Journal of Drug and Alcohol Abuse*, *38*(5), 498–504. https://doi.org/10.3109/00952990.2012.694530

Roberts, H., Jiles, R., Mokdad, A., Beckles, G., & Rios-Burrows, N. (2009). Trend analysis of diagnosed diabetes prevalence among American Indian/Alaska Native young adults–United States, 1994-2007. *Ethnicity & Disease, 19* (3), 276–279.

Robin, R. W., Chester, B., Rasmussen, J. K., Jaranson, J. M., & Goldman, D. (1997). Prevalence, characteristics, and impact of childhood sexual abuse in a southwestern American Indian tribe. *Child Abuse & Neglect*, *21*(8), 769–787. https://doi.org/10.1016/S0145-2134(97)00038-0

Salvail, F. R., & Smith, J. M. (2007). *Survey shows the Hawaii behavioral risk factor surveillance system special report*. Department of Health State of Hawaii. https://health.hawaii.gov/brfss/files/2013/11/PrevalenceOfAnxietyAndDepression.pdf

Siordia, C., Bell, R. A., & Haileselassie, S. L. (2017). Prevalence and risk for negative disability outcomes between American Indians-Alaskan Natives and other race-ethnic groups in the Southwestern United States. *Journal of Racial and Ethnic Health Disparities*, *4*(2), 195–200. https://doi.org/10.1007/s40615-016-0218-z

Stanley, L.R, Harness, S.D, Swaim, R.C, & Beauvais, F. (2014). Rates of substance use of american indian students in 8th, 10th, and 12th grades living on or near reservations: update, 2009-2012. *Public Health Reports*, 129(2), 156-163. doi. https://doi.org/10.1177/003335491412900209

Tipps, R. T., Buzzard, G. T., & McDougall, J. A. (2018). The opioid epidemic in Indian country. *The Journal of Law, Medicine & Ethics*, *46*(2), 422–436. https://doi.org/10.1177/1073110518782950

Urban Indian Health Institute. (2014). *Supporting sobriety among American Indians and Alaska Natives: A literature review, 2014.*

Urban Indian Health Institute. (2018). *Missing and murdered Indigenous women and girls: A snapshot of data from 71 urban cities in the United States* (Report No. 2- Our Bodies, Our Stories: Our work to advocate and provide data to protect Native women). http://www.uihi.org/wp-content/uploads/2018/11/Missing-and-Murdered-Indigenous-Women-and-Girls-Report.pdf

U.S. Census Bureau. (2010). Census CPH-T-6. American Indian and Alaska Native Tribes in the United States and Puerto Rico: 2010. Table 66. American Indian and Alaska Native Population by Tribe for Puerto Rico: 2010. Internet release date: December 2013. census.gov/population/www.cen2010/cph-t/t-6tables/Table%20(66).pdf

US Census. (2012a). *The American Indian and Alaska Native population: 2010*. (2010 Census Briefs). Jan. 12, 2012.

US Census. (2012b).*The native Hawaiian and other pacific Islander population: 2010*. (2010 Census Briefs). May 2, 2012.

US Department of Health and Human Services. (2013). *Child maltreatment 2012*. http://www.acf.hhs.gov/programs/cb/research-data-technology/statistics-research/child-maltreatment

Walters, K. L., Johnson-Jennings, M., Stroud, S., Rasmus, S., Charles, B., & Boulafentis, J. (2020). Growing from our roots: Strategies for developing culturally grounded health promotion interventions in American Indian, Alaska Native, and Native Hawaiian communities. *Prevention Science*, *21*(Suppl 1), 54–64. https://doi.org/10.1007/s11121-018-0952-z

Walters, K. L., Mohammed, S. A., Evans-Campbell, T., Beltrán, R. E., Chae, D. H., & Duran, B. (2011). Bodies don't just tell stories, they tell histories: Embodiment of historical trauma among American Indians and Alaska Natives. *Dubois Review*, *8*(1), 179–189. https://doi.org/10.1017/S1742058X1100018X

Walters, K. L., Stately, A., Evans-Campbell, T., Simoni, J. M., Duran, B., Schultz, K., . . . Guerrero, D. (2009). "Indigenist" collaborative research efforts in Native American communities. In A. R. Stiffman (Ed.) The Field Research Survival Guide, pp. 146–173. New york, NY: Oxford University Press.

Welty, T. K., Rhoades, D. A., Yeh, F., Lee, E. T., Cowan, L. D., Fabsitz, R. R., Robbins, D. C., Devereux, R. B., Henderson, J. A., & Howard, B. V. (2002). Changes in cardiovascular disease risk factors among American Indians: The strong heart study. *Annals of Epidemiology*, *12*(2), 97–106. https://doi.org/10.1016/S1047-2797(01)00270-8

Wexler, L., Silveira, M. L., & Bertone-Johnson, E. (2012). Factors associated with Alaska Native fatal and nonfatal suicidal behaviors 2001–2009: Trends and implications for prevention. *Archives of Suicide Research*, *16*(4), 273–286. https://doi.org/10.1080/13811118.2013.722051

Whitbeck, L. B., Walls, M. L., Johnson, K. D., Morrisseau, A. D., & McDougall, C. M. (2009). Depressed affect and historical loss among North American Indigenous adolescents. *American Indian and Alaska Native Mental Health Research*, *16*(3), 16. https://doi.org/10.5820/aian.1603.2009.16

White, A., Richardson, L. C., Li, C., Ekwueme, D. U., & Kaur, J. S. (2014). Breast cancer mortality among American Indian and Alaska Native women, 1990–2009. *American Journal of Public Health*, *104*(S3), S432–S438. https://doi.org/10.2105/AJPH.2013.301720

Yuan, N. P., Belcourt-Dittloff, A., Schultz, K., Packard, G., & Duran, B. M. (2015). Research agenda for violence against American Indian and Alaska Native women: Toward the development of strength-based and resilience interventions. *Psychology of Violence*, *5*(4), 367–373. https://doi.org/10.1037/a0038507

Zamora-Kapoor, Z., Nelson, L., Barbosa-Leiker, C., Comtois, K., Walker, L., & Buchwald, D. (2016). Suicidal ideation in American Indian/Alaska Native and White adolescents: The role of social isolation, exposure to suicide, and overweight. *American Indian and Alaska Native Mental Health Research: Journal of the National Center*, 23, 86–100.

Part 1

Promotive, Protective, and Risk Factors for Indigenous Health Equity

A culturally informed scoping review of Native Hawaiian mental health and emotional well-being literature

Rachel L. Burrage[iD], Matilda M. Antone, Kristin N. M. Kaniaupio, and Kira L. Rapozo

ABSTRACT

The need for culturally grounded research on Native Hawaiian (NH) mental health and psychological well-being has been discussed by practitioners and researchers for more than four decades. This study combines scoping review methodology with culturally informed inclusion criteria in order to identify and synthesize literature on NH mental health and psychological well-being that is grounded in NH understandings of well-being. A systematic search of peer-reviewed literature and doctoral dissertations that linked NH mental health and psychological well-being to physical, social, spiritual, or cultural factors produced 81 studies. Twenty-one studies that were methodologically framed in NH culture were then selected for data extraction. These studies emphasized the importance of family, spirituality, connection to place, and cultural identity for mental and emotional well-being, as well as the inclusion of culture in interventions.

Evidence suggests that Native Hawaiian (NH) people prefer and find more satisfaction in traditional healing methods than in Euro-Western clinical approaches to mental health (Bell et al., 2001; Park et al., 2018). At the same time, NH people have lower rates of mainstream mental health service use when compared with other ethnic groups (Ta et al., 2008). Such trends are possibly attributable to differences in conceptualizations of health and well-being between NH culture and Euro-Western models of well-being. This is troubling, as NH people also exhibit higher rates than other ethnic groups in Hawai'i on many indicators of psychological distress, including depression, suicide, and anxiety (Andrade et al., 2006; Hawaii Health Data Warehouse, 2014).

Unlike in Euro-Western traditions, where mental health is largely considered a property of an individual, there is no single equivalent concept in traditional NH understandings of well-being. NH conceptualizations of self extend beyond the individual, and are intricately linked to society and the natural world. As such the concept of lōkahi[1] or harmony between kanaka (humankind), 'āina (the land), and ke akua (god or gods) is central to NH understandings of well-being. McGregor et al. (2003) propose an ecological model of NH well-being that centers the individual in the 'ohana or extended as the basic social unit. Well-being at this level does not only include the present family system; it also involves the past, through connections to ancestors that involve land and genealogy, and connection to future through transmission of culture, language, and ways of knowing and being. Other authors note that personal well-being from a NH view point is holistic in nature and encompasses the physical, mental, and spiritual domains, in which the physical refers to both an individual's physical body and a connection to land (McCubbin & Marsela, 2009; Mokuau, 2011)

Okamoto, Kulis, Marsiglia, Holleran Steiker, and Dustman (2014) define culturally grounded interventions as those that are created "from the ground up" and center the culture and social context of a particular population. Calls for culturally grounded research on NH mental health have been made since the mid 1980s (Native Hawaiian Health Research Consortium [NHHRC], 1985) and continue today (Kūkulu Kumuhana Planning Committee, 2017). As such, there is a need not only to ground future research in NH culture but to understand what culturally grounded research already exists regarding NH mental health and well-being. This review seeks to synthesize the literature on Native Hawaiian mental health and psychological well-being by conducting a culturally informed review in order to produce a literature review that is grounded in NH understandings of well-being.

Creating a "culturally informed" review of literature

Like many research methodologies, the literature review is a cultural construct. It at once synthesizes empirical knowledge and, in the process, assesses the value of that knowledge based on a specific set of criteria. Two of the most common methodologies for the synthesis of empirical research are the *systematic review* and the *scoping review*, although many other methodologies exist (see Kastner et al., 2016 for a detailed discussion). The "gold standard" of these is the Cochrane systematic review, which is focused on synthesizing clinical trials and places a great deal of attention on evaluating the validity of studies through close attention to their experimental designs (Higgins & Green, 2011). However, as Kirmayer (2012) notes, the type of knowledge synthesized in systematic reviews and the type of knowledge valued by many Indigenous communities represent different epistemological cultures; bringing together research and Indigenous communities requires flexibility in what are considered to be valid types of knowledge construction.

An alternative to the systematic review is the scoping review. The scoping review is a flexible, exploratory methodology that seeks to synthesize a broad array of evidence on a particular topic. Like the systematic review, scoping reviews involve a research question, a systematic search to identify relevant studies, the selection of studies based on specific inclusion and exclusion criteria, and the eventual charting, summarizing, and reporting of results (Colquhoun et al., 2014). Unlike systematic reviews, inclusion and exclusion criteria for scoping reviews may be developed *ad hoc*, using an iterative process as articles are reviewed; the results are often compared qualitatively, with less attention to study quality (Armstrong et al., 2011). Although a scoping review is more flexible in its inclusion and valuation of different types of knowledge, it still represents a Euro-Western tradition of knowledge creation through empirical research. For example, simply limiting search criteria to a specified date range excludes important primary sources of traditional knowledge that may represent NH understandings of well-being. Unlike in Euro-Western understandings, ancestral knowledge does not necessarily have an expiration date.

Still, steps can be taken to make sure that a scoping review is as inclusive of NH understandings of well-being as possible. For example, current research that is grounded in NH culture may not use mainstream Euro-Western constructs or measures related to mental health. Culturally grounded research may use Hawaiian constructs such as 'ohana (family), 'āina (land) or lōkahi (balance), or measures of psychological well-being such as self-esteem that may not normally be considered as mental health outcomes. The current review follows Colquhoun (2014) to conduct a scoping review on NH mental health and well-being. It incorporates three strategies for cultural informing: a) amplifying the search strategy to include terms for psychological well-being that might not normally be considered part of the mental health literature, b) narrowing selection criteria to include only studies that examine holistic relationships between different types of well-being, and c) specifically examining studies that are methodologically grounded in NH culture or identity.

Method

Research team

The research team consisted of one non-Indigenous faculty member and three Native Hawaiian women undergraduate research assistants, all non-traditional students. The non-Indigenous faculty member had over ten years of clinical, community, and research experience working with Indigenous communities in continental United States and had previously contributed to two systematic reviews on Indigenous psychological well-being (Gone et al., 2019; Pomerville, Burrage, & Gone, 2016). All three research assistants were seniors in a Bachelor of Social Work program at the time of writing and had previously participated in the Native Hawaiian Interdisciplinary Health Program, a semester-long place-based learning course focused on Native Hawaiian ways of knowing and healing. The first research assistant had both professional and personal experience working Native Hawaiian kūpuna (elders) and keiki (children), including having had the privilege to develop strong relationships with kūpuna in the community of Kalaupapa on the island of Moloka'i. The second research assistant was raised in Kalihi on the island of O'ahu, a community heavily influenced by Native Hawaiian and several other Pacific Island cultures, and has specific interests related to the impacts of a cancer diagnosis for Native Hawaiian families. The third research assistant was born and raised on the island of Kaua'i, and is a haumana (student) of la'au lapa'au (Hawaiian natural medicine), with an interest in integrating Native Hawaiian practices into therapeutic mental health settings to promote health and wellness in NH communities.

Search strategy

Given that Native Hawaiian understandings of well-being incorporate physical, mental, spiritual, and relational well-being, the research team decided to focus on intersections of NH mental health and psychological well-being with physical, spiritual, and relational concepts. A science and technology reference librarian who was trained in systematic reviews and familiar with scoping review methodology was consulted for this project. Additionally, a reference librarian specializing in Native Hawaiian studies was consulted for sources of Hawaiian Language terms that broadly reflect well-being or healing practices. Hawaiian language search terms were drawn from *Nānā I Ke Kumu* (Pukui et al., 1979) a glossary designed for health professionals with information on Native Hawaiian understandings of health, and the *Report of the E Ola Mau Task Force* (E Ola Mau, The Native Health Consortium, 1985), a statewide assessment on Native Hawaiian health.

Search terms related to Native Hawaiians (e.g. "Native Hawaiian," "Kanaka Maoli," or "Pacific Islander") as well as search terms related to psychosocial well-being or mental illness (e.g. mental, cognitive, wellness, depression, quality-of-life, stress, trauma, resilience) or Hawaiian language terms (e.g. lōkahi, laulima, 'ohana, piko, ho'oponopono, lomilomi) were then used to search titles and abstracts for journal articles and dissertations since the year 2000 in the following databases: PsycINFO, PsycARTICLES, Social Services Abstracts, Social Work Abstracts, PubMed, CINAHL, ProQuest Dissertations and Theses, Proquest Dissertations and Theses at the University of Hawaii, Web of Science, Social Sciences, and Emerging Sources citation indices. The full list of search terms is available upon request. After removing duplicates, this search produced 2,468 results.

Screening and data extraction

Three criteria were used to determine whether to include an article in this study. The article had to be a) an empirical study b) about Native Hawaiians in either Hawai'i or the mainland United States and c) link psychological well-being to relational, physical, spiritual, or cultural constructs. For the first criteria, studies were excluded that were either review papers, including systematic reviews, or were only theoretical in nature. Second, studies were only included if all participants self-identified as Native Hawaiians or results were disaggregated by ethnicity. Most of the studies excluded under this criterion combined NH with other Pacific Islanders or Asians, although some were excluded because they included non-NH family members of NH people and did not disaggregate the results. Finally, studies had to examine the link between psychological well-being and either physical, relational, spiritual, or other cultural constructs. Figure 1 summarizes the full screening and data extraction process.

Psychological well-being was defined broadly as anything relating to cognitive, emotional, or mental health. Substance use or abuse was excluded due to the existence of a prior review on this topic (Edwards et al., 2010). Conditions with clear neurological underpinnings, such as neurodevelopmental and neurocognitive disorders were also excluded. Physical constructs were defined as anything relating to physical health and wellness. Social constructs were defined as anything that included relations with other people or social context, such as sociodemographic variables. Spiritual factors were defined as anything having to do with relationship to god(s), religious or spiritual practices or beliefs. Cultural factors included NH healing practices, cultural practices, and NH identity or cultural affiliation.

The titles and abstracts of the data corpus were divided into two groups, which were independently reviewed by two authors each to see if they met inclusion criteria. Each pair of authors met to go over discrepancies in their decisions. In the case that the authors were unable to reach an agreement as to whether to include or exclude a particular article, the article was brought to the full research team for discussion and clarification. Of the 2,468 articles reviewed, 10 had to be discussed by the full research team to see if they met criteria for inclusion. This first round of screening produced 81 results.

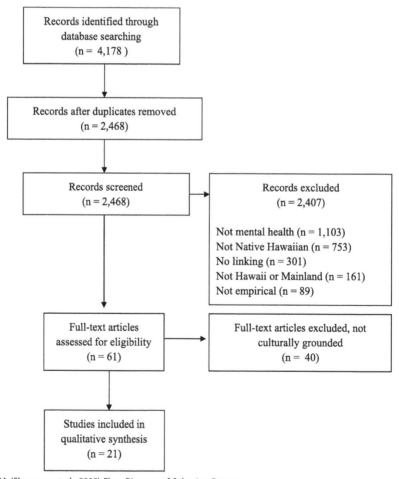

Figure 1. PRISMA (Shamseer et al., 2005) Flow Diagram of Selection Process.

A team of three authors then reviewed the full text of these articles to determine whether they met additional two selection criteria: a) Was the study framed or grounded in NH cultural concepts, values, or practices? and/or b) Did the study use a measure of NH culture or identity? As in the previous round, a second member of the team also reviewed the documents for agreement. Once these additional criteria were applied, a total of 21 articles met one or both criteria for inclusion in this study. The full text of these articles was then reviewed in order to extract data concerning their methods and conclusions.

Results

The 21 selected studies are summarized in Table 1. In the case where studies included non-NH participants, only the NH participants are noted in the table. The topics of these papers can be divided into several categories: a) the importance of 'ohana and social connection in overcoming adversity; b) connection between cultural identity and mental health; c) incorporation of Hawaiian culture into interventions; and d) connection to place and mental or emotional health.

The importance of 'ohana and social connections in overcoming adversity

Of the 21 studies included in this review, seven of them drew conclusions about the importance of support from 'ohana (family) or other social connections for well-being when overcoming adversity.

Mokuau and Braun (2007) examined how family support and dynamics affect NH women living with breast cancer. This study utilized focus groups as a means to integrate oral-aural tradition into the research methodology, an important component of NH culture. Each focus group meeting began with pule (prayer) led by a kūpuna (elder) as this was culturally relevant to NH culture and protocol. The results of this study showed that NH women living with breast cancer relied on 'ohana (family), ho'omana (spirituality), and kōkua (assistance). A second study utilizing the same methodology examined NH women's experiences with breast cancer from diagnosis through recovery. The results of this study showed that religion, spirituality, and giving back to others (kōkua) were vital for survivors in order to persevere during their cancer journey (Braun et al., 2002). Similarly, Calumet (2017) conducted phone interviews to study the importance of mana'olana (hope) in dealing with a cancer diagnosis. Results showed that families help to generate hope for cancer patients, which appeared to impact how a patient perceived their overall physical and mental state. Results of this study also showed that when breast cancer survivors shared their cancer journey with others, it reaffirmed a sense of hope and joy.

Shahan (2009) explored various diabetes disparities between Whites and NH adults using the Behavioral Risk Factor Surveillance System. This study used a decolonization framework, incorporating NH cultural and historical context and understanding of illness and healing into the interpretation of its results. Results revealed that social and emotional support had a greater impact in predicting sense of general health for NH with diabetes than for Whites with diabetes. In another comparative study, Anngela-Cole and Busch (2011) examined the relationship between stress, anticipatory mourning, and cultural practices amongst caregivers of family members with terminal cancer. They found that Native Hawaiians had unique ways of coping with stress and anticipatory mourning when compared with Chinese, Japanese, and European Americans. These included a perception of lower stress due to the fact that caregiving was normal in intergenerational households, and that the entire family was expected to provide care. NH people also expressed a reliance on god and prayer, as well as the understanding that ancestors were a part of the family and families remained unified even after the passing of a loved one.

Goebert et al. (2000) compared Hawaiian and non-Hawaiian students' self-reports of mental health, family environment, major life events, support from family and friends, Hawaiian cultural identity, and suicide. The results of this study showed that Hawaiian adolescents experienced significantly more adversity than non-Hawaiian adolescents. Family adversity had a greater effect on psychiatric symptoms than any other factor. However, family support also reduced the risk for internalizing symptoms, particularly for Hawaiian adolescents, showing the importance of family

Table 1. Descriptions of studies included in scoping review.

Authors	Type	Data Source	n	Geography	Age	Sex	Population	Psychological Construct	Linking Construct	Linking Construct (Detail)	Conclusions
Andres (2002)	Article	Interviews	4	Oʻahu	42–74	75% female	Hakus (Hoʻoponopono practitioners)	Sense of safety; Emotional expression; Positive feelings; Aloha	Social; Spiritual; Cultural	Prayer; Cultural groundedness;	Sense of safety; emotional expression, and aloha were important part of the practice, together with spiritual and family components. Conducting hoʻoponopono also lead to positive feelings for practitioners.
Anngela-Cole and Busch (2011)	Article	Focus groups	12	Oʻahu	M = 57	83.33% female	Caregivers	Stress Anticipatory grief	Social; Spiritual	Family support; Belief in god/prayer	Social and spiritual factors may explain lower caregiving stress.
Bell et al. (2001)	Article	Survey	285	Statewide	Adolescents	Not stated for NH	High school students	Mental health; Identity	Culture	Use of traditional healers	Mental health did not predict healer use among NH adolescents, but cultural identity did.
Braun et al. (2002)	Article	Focus groups	45	Oʻahu and neighbor islands	36–80 (M = 58)	80% female	Cancer survivors	Cancer survival (coping); Personal strength, perseverance	Social; spiritual	Family support; Spirituality; Helping others	Participants were sustained through cancer through personal strength and perseverance, helping others, support from others, and spiritual support.
Browne and Braun (2017)	Article	Interviews and focus groups	30	U.S. Mainland	Varied by data source	Not stated	Older adults and caregivers	Stress	Culture; social	Poverty; Discrimination; Stigma; Ties to Hawaiʻi	Respondents reported stressors related to leaving Hawaiʻi as well as being distant from Hawaiʻi.
Browne et al. (2014).	Article	Listening sessions	24 kūpuna; 17 caregivers	Hawaiʻi, Molokaʻi, Kauaʻi, primarily rural	Kūpuna: 60 to 95 (M = 77) Caregivers: 38–77 (M = 57)	Kūpuna: 87.5% female Caregivers: 64.71% female	Kūpuna and caregivers	Emotional well-being; Coping	Cultural; Spiritual	Prayer and spirituality; Cultural foods	Prayer, spirituality, kalo, and poi were considered important for emotional well-being and coping.
Calumet (2017)	Dissertation	Interviews	5	California	47–74 (M = 62)	Women	Breast cancer patients	Manaʻolana (hope)	Social; Spiritual; Physical	Family support; Support group; Religion/ relationship with God; Nature	Social and spiritual factors contributed to hope, which improved breast cancer journey.

(Continued)

Table 1. (Continued).

Authors	Type	Data Source	n	Geography	Age	Sex	Population	Psychological Construct	Linking Construct	Linking Construct (Detail)	Conclusions
Carlton et al. (2006)	Article	Secondary analysis	1832	Not stated	Not stated for NH	Not stated for NH	High school students	Psychiatric symptomology; Optimism	Social; physical; cultural	Family support; Family adversity; Physical health; Hawaiian language and sovereignty	Family support, physical fitness and health, and optimism significantly contributed to well-being for internalizing symptoms. Achievement, physical fitness and health, and family support significantly contributed to well-being based on externalizing symptoms. Hawaiian language and Hawaiian sovereignty were significantly associated with decreased well-being.
Goebert et al. (2000)	Article	Survey	2634	3 islands, suburban and rural	Adolescents	Not stated	High school students	Psychiatric symptomology	Social	Family social support; family adversity	Family adversity was associated with increased symptomology; family support reduced risk, with low support having a greater impact on internalizing symptomology for NH youth than for non-NH youth.
Kaholokula et al. (2012)	Article	Survey	146	Hawai'i island, rural	18 and over	71.23% female	Men and nonpregnant women	Stress	Social; cultural	Racism; Cultural affiliation;	Increased attributed racism was linked to lower levels of cortisol when controlling for other factors.
Kuikahi-Duncan (2016)	Dissertation	Mixed Methods	102	O'ahu	Not stated for NH	Not stated for NH	Community college students	Depression; anxiety	Cultural	Cultural blendedness; Cultural harmony	Native Hawaiians who reported high levels of cultural blendedness reported high levels of depressive symptoms.
Kuratani (2015)	Dissertation	Interviews	29	O'ahu	24–88 (M = 56)	55% female	General	Warm feelings/ comfort; Empathy; Identity	Cultural	Food; land access	Access to food and land is linked to identity, and traditional foods contribute to comfort and empathy through cooking and sharing
McCubbin (2003)	Dissertation	Survey	243	O'ahu	Not stated	Not stated	10th and 11th grade private school students	Stress; Depression; Anxiety; Self-acceptance; Personal growth	Social; cultural	Native Hawaiian Stress; Ethnic identity;	Ethnic identity was negatively correlated with depression, and positively correlated with Native Hawaiian stress, self-acceptance, and personal growth.

(Continued)

Table 1. (Continued).

Authors	Type	Data Source	n	Geography	Age	Sex	Population	Psychological Construct	Linking Construct	Linking Construct (Detail)	Conclusions
McMullin (2005)	Article	Participant observation; interviews	36	Hawai'i and Maui	20–86	Not stated	General	Emotional life; Stress; Positive attitude; Confidence	Physical; spiritual	Balance	Respondents viewed health as a balance between physical, spiritual, and emotional life, and also resulting from low stress, a positive attitude, and confidence.
Mokuau and Braun (2007)	Article	Focus groups	8	Not stated	43–84 (M = 68)	Women	Breast cancer patients	Emotional support	Social; Spiritual	Family support; Church/ spirituality	Family and church/spirituality were reported as contributors to emotional support by breast cancer patients.
Mokuau et al. (2012)	Article	RCT	29	O'ahu, Hawai'i, Moloka'i	50's	Women	Breast cancer patients	Self-efficacy; Coping;	Cultural	Culturally tailored intervention	Culturally-tailored intervention improved self-efficacy and coping as compared to control group.
Oneha (2000)	Dissertation	Interviews; participant observation; photography	13	O'ahu, rural	36–80	61.52% female	General	General well-being; Pono (balance of mind, body, spirit) Comfort and safety Feeling of belonging	Cultural; Spiritual	Sense of place	Sense of place was intricately tied to well-being, feelings of belonging, a sense of comfort and safety, spiritual connections to ancestors, and pono (health through a balance of mind, body, or spirit).
Roberts and Hitchcock (2018)	Article	Focus groups	103	Hawai'i island	Not stated	Not stated	11th &12th grade, college freshmen, college sophomores	Self-efficacy Aspiration	Cultural	Cultural identity; Cultural practices.	Having culturally appropriate mentoring for college prep, including a focus on identity, helped improve student self-efficacy and aspirations.
Scanlan (2013)	Dissertation	Web-based survey	184	Nationwide	18–60 (M = 27.11)	73.8% female	College Students	Depression; Anxiety; Psychological distress; Psychological well-being	Culture	Cultural affiliation; Cultural congruence	Cultural variables had a positive impact on psychological well-being, mediated by anxiety and depression.
Shahan (2009)	Dissertation	Secondary analysis	138	Statewide	Not stated for NH	Not stated for NH	Individuals diagnosed with diabetes	Social and emotional support; Life satisfaction	Physical	General health; Diabetes management	The interaction of socioemotional support and race predicted general health, as did life satisfaction among Native Hawaiians.
Yuen et al. (2000)	Article	Survey	2237	Statewide	Not stated for NH	Not stated for NH	High school students	Suicidality	Cultural	Cultural identity	Hawaiian cultural identity was positively correlated with suicide risk, but may be due to correlation between identity and ethnicity.

support and cultural identity for psychological well-being. Similarly, Carlton et al. (2006) compared multiple indicators of resilience, family adversity, and well-being between NH and non-NH youth. Family support, physical fitness, and health contributed to well-being for both internalizing and externalizing symptoms for NH youth; however, Hawaiian language and sovereignty indicators were negatively associated with well-being.

Connection between cultural identity and mental health

Six of the articles found in this review examined the relationship between cultural identity and mental health, five using survey methods and one using qualitative interviews.

Using a web-based survey, Scanlan (2013) examined the relationship between cultural affiliation, campus cultural congruence, and anxiety, depression, and psychological well-being among Native Hawaiian college participants. Findings suggested that cultural variables play a positive role in psychological well-being. Native Hawaiian students who endorsed higher cultural affiliation also reported experiencing fewer symptoms of depression and anxiety. Similarly, McCubbin (2003) found that Hawaiian ethnic identity was negatively correlated with depression, and positively correlated with self-acceptance and personal growth among Native Hawaiian students at a private high school.

In contrast, Kuikahi-Duncan (2016) examined the relationship between bicultural identity integration, depression, anxiety, and academic achievement in Native Hawaiian community college students on Oahu using questionnaires. Students with higher scores of Bicultural Identity Integration reported higher depressive and anxiety symptoms. A negative relationship between psychological well-being and different measures of Hawaiian culture or identity was also found by Carlton et al. (2006), as previously discussed. One possible explanation for this, provided by Yuen et al. (2000), is that there is a high inter-correlation between identity and ethnicity. Although these authors found that suicidality was positively correlated with Native Hawaiian cultural identity, they noted that it may be due to the relationship between identity and ethnicity. Kaholokula et al. (2012) examined correlations between perceived racism and physiological stress in Native Hawaiians by measuring cortisol activity and blood pressure. Participants completed a Hawaiian Cultural Identity scale, American Cultural Identity scale, Oppression Questionnaire, and Perceived Stress Scale. The results of the study concluded that there was an inverse correlation between attributed racism and cortisol levels among Native Hawaiians when controlling for socioeconomic, psychological, and biological factors. The authors suggested that this may be related to a blunting of hypothalamic pituitary adrenal (HPA) activity in the brain, which other studies have shown to be the result of prolonged stress exposure.

Finally, McMullin (2005) used participant observation and interviews on the islands of Maui and Hawaii to examine what it means to be a "healthy Hawaiian" by looking at culturally grounded themes that emphasize the importance of land, Hawaiian cultural identity and how it connects to NH spiritual, cultural, and overall well-being. The authors concluded that health, healing, and overall well-being in this scenario are achieved by reestablishing a tie between the land, Hawaiian ancestors, and a Hawaiian cultural identity.

Incorporation of Hawaiian culture into interventions

Four studies examined the incorporation of Hawaiian culture into interventions. Bell et al. (2001) examined treatment preferences for physical and mental health among NH and non-NH adolescents. For NH adolescents, increased Hawaiian cultural identity was associated with preference for use of Hawaiian healing practices, which are strongly rooted in spirituality and the connection between the mind, body, and soul. Adolescents that were strongly rooted in Hawaiian culture were more likely to prefer Hawaiian healing over conventional medicine, which tends to be more disease oriented. Similarly, Roberts and Hitchcock (2018) examined the impact of "culturally aligned" mentors on high school students. These supports were Native Hawaiian adults who mentored students in college preparation and included a focus on Native Hawaiian culture and practices. Although the focus of the intervention was college preparation, participants reported an increased sense of Hawaiian identity in addition to improved self-efficacy and aspirations for college and career.

Andres (2002) conducted interviews with practitioners of the Native Hawaiian peacemaking process of ho'oponopono, which is inclusive of the physical, emotional, and spiritual well-being of an individual in relationship to family, community, and the environment. Practitioners stated that a sense of safety, emotional expression, and aloha were all important parts of the practice; they also reported that conducting ho'oponopono lead to positive feelings for practitioners. A fourth study tested the cultural adaptation of psychoeducational materials to NH women coping with breast cancer using a randomized controlled trial. The waitlist control of women received basic information related to breast cancer, while the intervention group's sessions incorporated pule (prayer), kukakuka (talk story), and a focus on mea'ai (healthy eating). At the end of fourth month, women in the culturally adapted intervention group had made statistically significant improvements in self-efficacy and coping, while the control group had not (Mokuau et al., 2012).

Connection to place and mental or emotional health

Four studies explored connections between physical environment and mental or emotional well-being. In one study, 13 Native Hawaiian men and women of various adult ages from the Waianae coast of Oahu were interviewed about their sense of place (Oneha, 2000). Each participant was invited to speak freely using language that was most comfortable for them. They discussed how their cultural lands had impacted the way they treated others in the community, how they perceived their personal identity, and how the land contributed to their physical, mental, and spiritual health. Most of the participants communicated that they felt they were part of the land, and that the land was part of them; therefore, they could not be separated in order for one another to exist.

Browne et al. (2014) examined social and health disparities faced by kūpuna and their 'ohana (family) caregivers in Hawai'i. Participants spoke about prayer and spirituality as coping mechanisms for the emotional well-being of both kūpuna and family caregivers. Participants also discussed the importance of kalo (taro) and poi (a dish made from taro) for physical, emotional, and spiritual health; they referred to kalo as being their medicine and poi having a spiritual connection. Another study by Browne and Braun (2017) examined resilience among Native Hawaiian kūpuna and their caregivers in California, away from the islands of Hawai'i. Some of the participants felt uneasy about their children being raised in "American culture," which would create a loss of their Native Hawaiian identities. Caregivers and kūpuna found also found it difficult to find Native Hawaiian health-care providers in California when seeking emotional and financial support for caregiving, making it harder to establish a trusting relationship with those that provided these services. Although these kūpuna and their 'ohana may have lost their physical connection to their lands, they still acknowledged their responsibility to their families as central to their culture.

Kuratani (2015) also examined the role food plays in comfort and empathy for many Native Hawaiians. For many of the participants, when they spoke of food, it brought many fond memories to mind as food was an important factor in cultural traditions and gatherings. For others, food from the lands they lived on was important as it helped cultivate their Native Hawaiian identities. Lack of access to land was linked to a cycle of oppression, the stress of which impacted NH well-being and identity. As previously mentioned, McMullin (2005) also suggested that connection to land was particularly important for NH concepts of well-being.

Discussion

This scoping review synthesized research on Native Hawaiian mental health and psychological well-being, using a culturally informed approach and paying particular attention to studies that were culturally grounded. Results show that multiple studies provide evidence for the importance of family support, spirituality, culturally grounded intervention, and connection to place as important contributors to psychological well-being and mental health among NH people. Studies demonstrated mixed results with respect to the relationship between NH identity and cultural practices with psychological well-being and mental health. This may be due to differences in the measures used, as well as the populations studied, and the difficulty of differentiating between factors related to ethnic identity and factors related to cultural affiliation.

This study has a number of limitations. As previously mentioned, limiting the review to articles published in 2000 and beyond excluded many important primary sources related to NH well-being. Future studies might examine primary sources, such as monographs and Hawaiian language newspapers, to understand prior conceptualizations of these concepts. Additionally, this review was limited to studies whose participants identified as NH, or where results were disaggregated. However, Hawai'i is a multi-ethnic society, and many NH families are also multi-ethnic. Thus, some studies that were excluded could have still provided insight into NH mental health and psychological well-being even though not all of the voices in the studies were NH. Examples are McCubbin (2006), an excellent study on ethnic schema in NH families that interviewed mostly NH individuals, but included several non-NH family members, or Isaacs (2018), a study on the effects of an intervention grounded in NH culture that was tested on a group of participants from various ethnic groups. The included studies were also limited in the way they incorporated NH culture. Although many took a culturally grounded approach, some of the larger studies simply included measures of Native Hawaiian culture and identity without grounding their conceptual framework in NH culture or history.

Future research into NH mental health and well-being should continue to use research methods that incorporate NH cultural values, practices, and concepts, as well as factors such as NH culture and identity. Researchers seeking to conduct trials of evidence-based practices or prevention programs should also ask whether the outcomes they are using are congruent with factors that have already been demonstrated to be of importance to NH mental health and well-being. For example, rather than examine impacts on mental health diagnoses, they might include measures of self-efficacy, self-esteem, cultural identity, family connectedness, or connection to the land, which the research summarized here has suggested are connected to NH well-being. Finally, researchers conducting systematic or scoping reviews on literature related to other Indigenous communities should consider framing their searches and inclusion criteria in a way that is congruent with the epistemologies and understandings of those communities, rather than using a solely Euro-Western framework for the constructs that they wish to review.

Note

1. Hawaiian words are not italicized in this manuscript, as italicized words are reserved for foreign languages, and the Hawaiian language is not a foreign language in Hawai'i.

Acknowledgments

We would like to acknowledge librarians Kapena Shim and Patricia Brandes at the University of Hawai'i at Mānoa Hamilton Library for their assistance in designing the search for this review.

Disclosure statement

No potential conflict of interest was reported by the authors.

ORCID

Rachel L. Burrage ⓘD http://orcid.org/0000-0003-0143-1147

References

Andres, B. S. (2002). *A qualitative phenomenological analysis of the critical incidents in the Native Hawaiian peacemaking process of "ho'oponopono"* [Unpublished doctoral dissertation]. The Wright Institute.

Andrade, N. N., Hishinuma, E. S., McDermott Jr., J. F., Johnson, R. C., Goebert, D. A., Makini Jr., G. K., Bell, C. K. (2006). The National Center on Indigenous Hawaiian Behavioral Health Study of Prevalence of Psychiatric Disorders in Native Hawaiian Adolescents. *Journal of the American Academy of Child & Adolescent Psychiatry, 45*(1), 26–36

Anngela-Cole, L., & Busch, M. (2011). Stress and Grief Among Family Caregivers of Older Adults With Cancer: A Multicultural Comparison From Hawai'i. Journal of Social Work in End-of-Life & Palliative Care, 7(4),318-337.

Armstrong, R., Hall, B. J., Doyle, J., & Waters, E. (2011). 'Scoping the scope' of a cochrane review. *Journal of Public Health, 33*(1), 147–150. https://doi.org/10.1093/pubmed/fdr015

Bell, C. K., Goebert, D. A., Andrade, N. N., Johnson, R. C., McDermott, J. F., Hishinuma, E. S., Carlton, B. S., Waldron, J. A., Makini, G. K., & Miyamoto, R. H. (2001). Sociocultural factors influencing adolescent preference and use of Native Hawaiian healers. *Complementary Therapies in Medicine, 9*(4), 224–231. https://doi.org/10.1016/S0965-2299(02)90000-2

Braun, K. L., Mokuau, N., Hunt, G. H., Kaanoi, M., & Gotay, C. C. (2002). Supports and obstacles to cancer survival for Hawaii's native people. *Cancer Practice, 10*(4), 192–200. https://doi.org/10.1046/j.1523-5394.2002.104001.x

Browne, C. V., & Braun, K. L. (2017). Away from the islands: Diaspora's effects on Native hawaiian elders and families in California. *Journal of Cross-Cultural Gerontology, 32*(4), 395–411. https://doi.org/10.1007/s10823-017-9335-3

Browne, C. V., Mokuau, N., Lana, S., Kim, B. J., Higuchi, P., & Braun, K. L. (2014). Listening to the voices of Native Hawaiian elders and 'ohana caregivers: Discussions on aging, health, and care preferences. *Journal of Cross-Cultural Gerontology, 29*(2), 131–151. https://doi.org/10.1007/s10823-014-9227-8

Calumet, K. M. (2017). *Breast cancer, mana'olana/hope, and the experience of Native Hawaiian women* [Unpublished doctoral dissertation]. Walden University.

Carlton, B. S., Goebert, D. A., Miyamoto, R. H., Andrade, N. N., Hishinuma, E. S., Makini, G. K., Jr., Yuen, N. Y. C., Bell, C. K., McCubbin, L. D., Else, R. N., & Nishimura, S. T. (2006). Resilience, family adversity and well-being among Hawaiian and non-Hawaiian adolescents. *International Journal of Social Psychiatry, 52*(4), 291–308. https://doi.org/10.1177/0020764006065136

Colquhoun, H. L., Levac, D., O'Brien, K. K., Straus, S., Tricco, A. C., Perrier, L., Kastner, M., & Moher, D. (2014). Scoping reviews: Time for clarity in definition, methods, and reporting. *Journal of Clinical Epidemiology, 67*(12), 1291–1294. https://doi.org/10.1016/j.jclinepi.2014.03.013

E Ola Mau, The Native Health Consortium. (1985). *Native Hawaiian health needs study: Report of E Ola Mau task force on health needs of Native Hawaiians.* Alu Like, Inc.

Edwards, C., Giroux, D., & Okamoto, S. K. (2010). A review of the literature on Native Hawaiian youth and drug use: Implications for research and practice. *Journal of Ethnicity in Substance Abuse, 9*(3), 153–172. https://doi.org/10.1080/15332640.2010.500580

Goebert, D., Nahulu, L., Hishinuma, E., Bell, C., Yuen, N., Carlton, B., Andrade, N. N., Miyamoto, R., & Johnson, R. (2000). Cumulative effect of family environment on psychiatric symptomatology among multiethnic adolescents. *Journal of Adolescent Health, 27*(1), 34–42. https://doi.org/10.1016/S1054-139X(00)00108-7

Gone, J. P., Hartmann, W. E., Pomerville, A., Wendt, D. C., Klem, S. H., & Burrage, R. L. (2019). The impact of historical trauma on health outcomes for indigenous populations in the USA and Canada: A systematic review. American Psychologist, 74(1), 20. http://dx.doi.org/10.1037/amp0000338

Hawaii Health Data Warehouse (2014). Depressive disorder, for the State of Hawaii, for the aggregated years- 2011-2013, 2012-2014. Retrieved from http://hhdw.org/wp-content/uploads/BRFSS_Depression_AGG3_00002_2011.pdf

Higgins, J. P. T., & Green, S. (Eds.). (2011). *Cochrane handbook for systematic reviews of interventions* (Version 5.1.0). The Cochrane Collaboration. https://handbook-5-1.cochrane.orghttps://handbook-5-1.cochrane.org

Isaacs, P. M. (2008). Aloha 'āina: A Hawaiian garden intervention designed to plant the seeds of recovery in persons with severe and persistent mental illness [Unpublished doctoral dissertation]. University of Hawai'i at Mānoa]

Kaholokula, J. K., Grandinetti, A., Keller, S., Nacapoy, A. H., Kingi, T. K., & Mau, M. K. (2012). Association between perceived racism and physiological stress indices in Native Hawaiians. *Journal of Behavioral Medicine, 35*(1), 27–37. https://doi.org/10.1007/s10865-011-9330-z

Kastner, M., Antony, J., Soobiah, C., Straus, S. E., & Tricco, A. C. (2016). Conceptual recommendations for selecting the most appropriate knowledge synthesis method to answer research questions related to complex evidence. *Journal of Clinical Epidemiology, 73*, 43–49. https://doi.org/10.1016/j.jclinepi.2015.11.022

Kirmayer, L. J. (2012). Cultural competence and evidence-based practice in mental health: Epistemic communities and the politics of pluralism. Social Science & Medicine, 75(2),249-256.

Kuikahi-Duncan, K. (2016). *Bicultural identity integration among Native Hawaiian college students* [Unpublished doctoral dissertation]. Palo Alto University.

Kūkulu Kumuhana Planning Committee. (2017). *Creating radical and new knowledge to improve Native Hawaiian wellbeing.* Lili'uokalani Trust.

Kuratani, D. L. G. (2015). *How do Native Hawaiian concepts of well-being inform the meaning and social function of food?* [Unpublished doctoral dissertation]. University of California, Los Angeles.

McCubbin, L. D. (2003). *Resilience among Native Hawaiian adolescents: Ethnic identity, psychological distress and well-being* [Unpublished doctoral dissertation]. The University of Wisconsin – Madison.

McCubbin, L. D. (2006). The role of Indigenous family ethnic schema on well-being among Native Hawaiian families. *Contemporary Nurse, 23*(2), 170–180. https://doi.org/10.5172/conu.2006.23.2.170

McCubbin, L. D., & Marsella, A. (2009). Native Hawaiians and psychology: The cultural and historical context of indigenous ways of knowing.. Cultural Diversity and Ethnic Minority Psychology, 15(4), 374.

McGregor, D. P., Morelli, P. T., Matsuoka, J. K., Rodenhurst, R., Kong, N., & Spencer, M. S. (2003). An ecological model of Native Hawaiian well-being. *Pacific Health Dialog, 10*(2), 106–128. https://pubmed.ncbi.nlm.nih.gov/18181424/

McMullin, J. (2005). The call to life: Revitalizing a healthy Hawaiian identity. *Social Science & Medicine, 61*(4), 809–820. https://doi.org/10.1016/j.socscimed.2004.08.051

Mokuau, N. (2011). Culturally based solutions to preserve the health of Native Hawaiians. *Journal of Ethnic & Cultural Diversity in Social Work, 20*(2), 98–113. https://doi.org/10.1080/15313204.2011.570119

Mokuau, N., & Braun, K. L. (2007). Family support for Native Hawaiian women with breast cancer. *Journal of Cancer Education, 22*(3), 191–196. https://doi.org/10.1007/BF03174336

Mokuau, N., Braun, K. L., & Daniggelis, E. (2012). Building family capacity for Native Hawaiian women with breast cancer. *Health & Social Work, 37*(4), 216–224. https://doi.org/10.1093/hsw/hls033

Native Hawaiian Health Research Consortium. (1985). *E ola mau: The Native Hawaiian health needs study: Medical task force report.* Alu Like, Inc.

Okamoto, S. K., Marsiglia, K. S., Holleran Steiker, F. F., & Dustman, L. K. (2014). A continuum of approaches toward developing culturally focused prevention interventions: From adaptation to grounding. *The Journal of Primary Prevention, 35*(2), 103–112. https://doi.org/10.1007/s10935-013-0334-z

Oneha, M. F. M. (2000). *Ka mauli O ka ʻāina a he mauli kānaka (the life of the land is the life of the people): An ethnographic study from a Hawaiian sense of place* [Unpublished doctoral dissertation]. University of Colorado Health Sciences.

Park, V. M. T., Kaholokula, J. K. A., Chao, P. J., & Antonio, M. (2018). Depression and help-seeking among Native Hawaiian women. *The Journal of Behavioral Health Services & Research, 45*(3), 454–468. https://doi.org/10.1007/s11414-017-9584-5

Pomerville, A., Burrage, R. L., & Gone, J. P. (2016). Empirical findings from psychotherapy research with indigenous populations: A systematic review. Journal of Consulting and Clinical Psychology, 84(12), 1023. https://doi.org/10.1037/ccp0000150

Pukui, M. K., Haertig, E. W., & Lee, C. A. (1979). *Nānā I Ke Kumu (Look to the Source) Volume I and Volume II.* Hui Hānai.

Roberts, K. D., & Hitchcock, C. H. (2018). Impact of culturally aligned supports on Native Hawaiian high school students' college attendance: A qualitative perspective. *Community College Journal of Research and Practice, 42*(4), 245–257. https://doi.org/10.1080/10668926.2017.1284698

Scanlan, K. R. L. (2013). *The relationship of cultural affiliation and cultural congruency to depression, anxiety, and psychological well-being among Native Hawaiian college students* [Unpublished doctoral dissertation]. Columbia University.

Shahan, K. M. (2009). *Health disparity in Native Hawaiians diagnosed with diabetes* [Unpublished doctoral dissertation]. Arizona State University.

Shamseer, L., Moher, D., Clarke, M., Ghersi, D., Liberati, A., Petticrew, M., Shekelle, P., & Stewart, L. A. (2005). Preferred reporting items for systematic review and meta-analysis protocols (PRISMA-P) 2015: Elaboration and explanation. *BMJ, 350*, g7647. https://doi.org/10.1136/bmj.g7647

Ta, V. M., Juon, H. S., Gielen, A. C., Steinwachs, D., & Duggan, A. (2008). Disparities in use of mental health and substance abuse services by Asian and Native Hawaiian/other Pacific Islander women. *The Journal of Behavioral Health Services & Research, 35*(1), 20–36.

Yuen, N. C. Y. C., Nahulu, L. B., Hishinuma, E. S., & Miyamoto, R. H. (2000). Cultural identification and attempted suicide in Native Hawaiian adolescents. *Journal of the American Academy of Child & Adolescent Psychiatry, 39*(3), 360–367. https://doi.org/10.1097/00004583-200003000-00019

What's love got to do with it? "Love" and alcohol use among U.S. Indigenous peoples: Aligning research with real-world experiences

Catherine E. McKinley ⓘ and Jenn Miller Scarnato ⓘ

ABSTRACT

This research examines how Indigenous families report experiences of love (a component of family resilience) and its association with the urgent health disparity of alcohol abuse. This exploratory mixed-methods study first identified emergent results from qualitative data ($n = 436$), which were then explored with follow-up quantitative data ($n = 127$) from a sample of Indigenous families in two Southeastern tribes. Love was a highly salient qualitative theme and component of family resilience. Quantitative results revealed cross-generational changes in family resilience, which were negatively associated with alcohol use. Current families may be transcending the effects of historical oppression by expressing love and family resilience.

Love is a highly salient concept in non-academic contexts that receives surprisingly little scholarly attention, despite its direct relevance to health and mental health equity. Moreover, how love might relate to important outcomes of interest such as alcohol use, is not well-understood. The purpose of this articles is to describe Indigenous participants' experiences of love, see how it varies across time and whether it relates in any systematic way to a primary health problem for many Indigenous peoples: alcohol use. Historically, the three varieties of love include (a) intimacy: feelings of closeness, warmth, and bonding; (b) passion: or sexual arousal and intensity; and (c) commitment: or the intentional choice to love and maintain that love with someone (Sternberg, 1986). Yet, this theory has primarily focused on love between romantic partners, rather than love within the broader family unit. This mismatch between the language used by the general population in comparison to the conceptualizations made by researchers marks a concerning incongruence between research and clinical practice. Indeed, the direct investigation of love is rarely included in health and mental health research; instead, love is broken down into its various conceptual elements, such as warmth and attachment, with little scholarly agreement on which conceptual elements best reflect how people experience love.

Although explicit attention to love is lacking, love is commonly operationalized in scholarly research as affection, bonding, warmth and comfort. Indeed, recent research has found that many conceptual elements associated with love promote mental health including parental bonding (Xu et al., 2018), family affection (León-del-Barco et al., 2018), and comfort and affection (Lowe et al., 2015), which were associated with positive mental health outcomes. Aspects of love were also found to be protective factors against suicidal ideation (Armstrong & Manion, 2015), juvenile offending (Barnert et al., 2015), and depression (Breton et al., 2015), lending further support for the clinical significance of love and its many dimensions. However, surprisingly little research has examined the influence of love on alcohol use and addictions. These are important areas of inquiry, especially among Indigenous peoples who experience a number of health and mental health disparities compared to the general U.S. population, including alcohol abuse (Whitbeck et al., 2004; Yu & Stiffman, 2007). A distinct trust responsibility by the federal government to provide for the health and well-being of 574 federally recognized tribes (Bureau of Indian Affairs, 2020), based on treaty agreements with politically sovereign tribes, makes this an urgent concern.

Alcohol abuse is a primary risk factor for Indigenous health disparities and is associated with the leading causes of death, such as cardiovascular disease (CVD) and diabetes (Chartier & Caetano, 2010; Thayer et al., 2017) as well as suicide (Masten & Monn, 2015; Sarche & Spicer, 2008; Tolan et al., 2006). Indigenous peoples tend to experience disproportionately high rates of alcohol abuse disorders, which drive increased mortality rates and are associated with family violence, including intimate partner violence (IPV) and child maltreatment (Bassuk et al., 2006; Masten & Monn, 2015; Tolan et al., 2006). Age-adjusted mortality rates for alcohol, chronic liver disease/cirrhosis among Indigenous peoples are 6.6 and 4.6 times higher than the general U.S. population, respectively.

According to the Framework of Historical Oppression, Resilience, and Transcendence (FHORT), historical oppression has undermined Indigenous communities and families through the imposition of historical traumas (e.g., boarding schools that stripped families' ability to socialize and transmit culture and language to their children), impairing the healthy transmission of affection and love and replacing such beliefs with antagonistic and oppressive social norms (Burnette, 2015). Consequently, social problems such as alcohol abuse and violence have increased; and, over time, these social ills may become internalized and normative, giving rise to various health disparities, such as substance abuse (Burnette, 2015). Despite being externally imposed, these problems may inadvertently become exacerbated and inter-generationally transmitted within Indigenous communities. Love, a core component of family resilience (the ability of families to overcome challenges) (Walsh, 2016) also relates to alcohol use.

Family tends to heavily influence substance use and health behaviors among Indigenous peoples (Burnette, 2017; Burnette & Figley, 2017; Martin & Yurkovich, 2014), making the connection between familial love and alcohol use a promising area for health disparities research. Because love is an integral part of family resilience, or the ability of families to bounce back and withstand adversity, this study examines the influence of love and family resilience on alcohol use, a leading precursor to health disparities amongst Indigenous peoples (Whitbeck et al., 2004; Yu & Stiffman, 2007).

This exploratory mixed-methods study begins with and prioritizes results from the qualitative component, and follows up with exploratory quantitative inquiry (Creswell, 2015). First, the lived experiences of love amongst Indigenous peoples are qualitatively analyzed, with an emphasis on love as a component of family resilience and strength. Second, quantitative analysis is used to examine intergenerational changes in expressions of love as a component of family resilience, measured by the Family Resilience Inventory (FRI), which includes items on verbal and physical expressions of love (Burnette et al., 2019). Third, the relationship between family resilience and alcohol use, a key health disparity among Indigenous peoples, is quantitatively examined. Rather than preemptively defining love, using the FHORT as a lens, through qualitative research this study reveals the perceptions and experiences of love amongst Indigenous peoples from two Southeastern tribes. We identify how love and family resilience may vary across generations, and how love, a key component of family resilience, relates to alcohol use.

Family love in cross-cultural contexts

Love is recognized as a fundamental human need that significantly impacts social and psychological well-being (Bauer, 2016; Gulledge et al., 2007; Noller, 1996; Riehl-Emde et al., 2003). Culture has been shown to influence the way that individuals experience a number of emotions, including love (Heshmati et al., 2017; Schmitt et al., 2009). Schmitt et al. (2009) observed cross-cultural variations in love in a quantitative study of 48 nations. Heshmati et al. (2017) found that, in addition to individual differences amongst people's perceptions of what it means to feel loved, cultural differences also greatly impact how love is expressed. Other research indicates cultural variations in perceptions and experiences of love (Karandashev, 2015).

In addition to cultural differences, love between family members is an important area of clinical focus, but a relatively neglected area of research. What limited research does investigate love tends to focus on intimate relationships, rather than whole family love (Graham, 2011; Riehl-Emde et al., 2003). Family love is believed to be affected by culture, and to have emotional, behavioral, and cognitive aspects (Noller, 1996) – all of which merit scholarly attention and clinical interest to enrich understandings of family resilience. Family resilience and support are integral for all family members, and can protect them from adverse outcomes and social problems that are often exacerbated due to the historical oppression of ethnic minorities (Burnette, 2016; 2017; 2019). Family resilience describes how the family collectively adapts to challenges and promotes family members' wellness and the wellness of the family as a whole (Masten & Monn, 2015). Family love is central to family resilience processes.

Studies of love amongst family members often focus on parental warmth and affection. Previous research has shown the value of physical and verbal affection in family systems, with particular attention to the influence of parental expressions of love on children's self-esteem and socio-emotional development (Sabey et al., 2018). Indeed, a review of the literature in this area revealed that physical affection within families positively impacts a variety of physical, social, and psychological outcomes (Gulledge et al., 2007) for family members. Moreover, in a systematic review specific to Indigenous peoples (Burnette & Figley, 2016), the quality of family relationships was a prominent theme predicting key behaviors related to Indigenous mental health and alcohol and other drug use disorders. Specifically, parental warmth, parental attachment, family support, caring, and communication were all found to play a protective role in abstaining from substance abuse amongst Indigenous young people (LaFromboise et al., 2006). This literature suggests that family love may play a protective role for Indigenous children and youth who might otherwise use alcohol and other substances, warranting further examination of the relationship between love, family resilience, and alcohol abuse to inform health and mental health interventions for Indigenous families. To our knowledge, this is the first study to examine this relationship.

Methods

This exploratory mixed-methods study places precedence on results from qualitative data, followed by a quantitative exploratory investigation (Creswell, 2015). A critical ethnography (study of culture that considers power dynamics in the analysis) was used to understand how family resilience and protective factors affect Indigenous peoples' alcohol abuse and well-being. The overarching research question was "What do Indigenous people see as the most important components of family resilience and strength?" Critical ethnographies prioritize the voices of participants, reporting results using language in participants' own words.

After qualitative data collection and analysis were complete, a survey was conducted to examine how themes identified in qualitative research (i.e., love and family resilience) predicted alcohol abuse outcomes, using a quantitative approach. This survey was administered to members of the same two Southeastern tribes that were sampled in the qualitative component of the study. Multiple forms of ethnographic data were collected from both tribes (existing, qualitative, and quantitative survey data) (Carspecken, 1996).

Setting

The inclusion of two tribes enabled the examination of universal themes and distinctions across populations. The identity of the tribes is kept confidential in line with tribal resolution agreements and as recommended by the Toolkit for Ethical and Culturally-Sensitive Research (Burnette, 2014). The "Inland Tribe" is a federally recognized tribe, whereas the "Coastal Tribe" is a state, but not federally recognized tribe. Recognition status influences the structure and resources of tribes immensely. The federally-recognized Inland Tribe provides tribal schooling, health services, social and family services, along with criminal justice and law enforcement. The state-recognized tribe provides programs for youth, and employment and educational programs. Both tribes have experienced severe historical oppression through educational discrimination, poverty, and racism.

Data collection

Recruitment efforts for all data (qualitative and quantitative) included word of mouth and disseminating fliers through Facebook, community agencies, tribal websites, and newsletters.

Qualitative

After tribal and IRB approval, data collection included: (a) participant observation; (b) individually-focused interviews; (c) family interviews; and (d) focus groups across the two tribes. Participant compensation for individual interviews and focus groups was a 20 USD gift card to a local department store, whereas compensation for family interviews was a 60 USD gift card for the whole family. Research questions derived from our research aims were developed into a semi-structured interview guide for focus groups and interviews. Following the methodological and cultural recommendations, individually-focused interviews took on a life history approach (Carspecken, 1996). Examples of probes from the semi-structured interview guide included: "What do you think is the most important thing about strong families? What keeps families strong? What is the 'glue' that holds families together? How do/did you know that you were cared for?" All participants who could be reached were given a copy of their individual life history interview, and wording was geared for 5th-grade comprehension-level.

Sample

A total of 436 participants were included across individually focused interviews, family interviews, and focus groups, with 228 Inland Tribe and 208 Coastal Tribe participants (See Table 1 for participant demographics). We gained perspectives from participants across the lifespan (elders, adults, and youth) in addition to professional perspectives from human service workers engaging tribal members. Individual interviews lasted, on average, 64 min minutes, whereas family interviews lasted, on average, 70 minutes; focus groups lasted, on average, 57 minutes.

Table 1. Participant Demographics and Sub-samples.

Types of Qualitative Data			
	Inland Tribe	**Coastal Tribe**	**Total**
Individually Focused	145	109	N=254
Family Focused	n=34 (80 participants)	n=30 (83 participants)	N=163 across 64 family interviews
Focus Groups	n=14 (113 participants)	n=13 (104 participants)	N=217 participants across 27 groups
Subsamples of Participants			
Subsample (n, %)	**Inland Tribe (N= 228)**	**Coastal Tribe (N= 208)**	**Total (N=436)**
Professional (18+)	47, 20.6%	23, 11.1%	70, 16.1%
Elder (56+)	44, 19.3%	61, 29.3%	105, 24.1%
Adult (24-55)	76, 33.3%	71, 34.1%	147, 33.7%
Youth (11-23)	61, 28.8%	53, 25.5%	114, 26.1%
Qualitative Data Participant Demographics			
	Inland Tribe (N= 228)	**Coastal Tribe (N= 208)**	**(N=436, 100%)**
Male	86, 37.7%	63, 30.3%	149, 33.9 %
Female	142, 62.3%	145, 69.7%	287, 65.8%
Married	62, 27.2%	64, 30.8%	126, 28.9 %
Number of children	2.53 (M)	2.57 (M)	2.55(M)
Number of siblings	4.81 (M)	4.61 (M)	4.70 (M)
Participant age (Mean)	37.1 (M)	42.5 (M)	39.7 (M)
Education	(n=149)	(n=158)	(N=307)
Less than high school	6	72	78, 25.4%
High school	33	36	69, 22.5%
Some college/vocational	53	16	69, 22.5%
Associates	31	16	47, 15.3%
Bachelors or higher	26	18	44, 14.3%
Quantitative Data Participant Demographics			
Secondary Data		**Inland Tribe, n=202**	**Coastal Tribe, n=293**
Quantitative Follow-Up Survey		Number (N=127)	Percent
Inland Tribe		80	63.0
Coastal Tribe		47	37.0
Male		23	19.1
Female		104	81.9

(*Continued*)

Table 1. (Continued).

Age	46.2 (*M*)	Range 21-80
Married	51	40.2
Number of children	3.77 (*M*)	*SD*=2.37
Less than high school	12	9.5
High school or equivalent	18	14.2
Some college/vocational	28	22.1
Associates	27	21.3
Bachelor's or higher	26	20.5
Working full-time	85	66.0
Somewhat difficult to pay bills/economically	69	54.3

Note. For group-based interviews (i.e., focus group and family interviews), total participants for each respective group are displayed in the row below total number of group interviews. The rows for age and number of children depict the average (*M*). Some participants participated in more than one type of interview. For educational attainment in the qualitative data, available/applicable data were less than the total, due to the inclusion of youth, who were still in high school

Quantitative

Participants completed a survey, delivered online through Qualtrics (Qualtrics, 2014). All survey participants were entered into a drawing for a 50 USD gift card with over half ($n = 70$, 55%) receiving this gift card. Participants' names were kept separately from data and collected only for compensation purposes. In total, 161 participants started the survey with 79% completing the survey ($n = 127$).

Data analysis

Qualitative

Collaborative and team-based data analysis methods were used given the extensive ethnographic data collected (Guest & MacQueen, 2008). All qualitative data were professionally transcribed before being transferred to NVivo software for analysis. To enhance cultural sensitivity, data analysis teams included Indigenous PhD students from each tribe and two non-Indigenous PhD students along with the first author. Reconstructive analysis, a specific method of thematic qualitative analysis, was used throughout, which involved: (a) immersion in transcripts multiple times, arriving at a holistic conception of data (b) creating hierarchical codes and sub-codes developed through consensus; and (c) in-depth analysis of implicit and explicit meanings. Interrater reliability was evaluated using Cohen's Kappa coefficients (McHugh, 2012), which were extremely high (.90 or above).

Unifying and culturally-specific themes are identified by indicating the tribe in the results for reference. The theme "love" was coded across 95 sources and referenced 158 times. Broken down by tribe, this theme was spoken about by 48 Inland Tribe sources (i.e., individual interviews, family interviews, and focus groups) and referenced 76 times, and by 47 Coastal Tribe sources and referenced 82 times. The sub-themes identified for this article are those related to love that most frequently occurred across tribes. Regarding gender breakdown, for the Inland Tribe, themes were reported across 39 female participants and 15 male participants, four focus groups, and eleven family interviews. For the Coastal Tribe, themes were reported across 44 female participants and 14 male participants, two focus groups, and nine family interviews.

Rigor

Meeting the standards of rigor for this particular method (Carspecken, 1996), each participant who was reachable received a summary of the results, copies of the interview, survey information, and opportunities to make any changes to the interview transcript or results (i.e., member-checks). No participants disagreed with interpretations, and many extended and elaborated upon results. Results were disseminated to tribes on more than 10 occasions by providing trainings, along with tribal agency, tribal council, and community group presentations and community dialogue groups. Weekly debriefing took place across research team members, and 'consistency checks' ensured participants' explanations were congruent with what was reported. Multiple participants (55.5%) were interviewed more than one time.

Quantitative

Qualitative results informed the emergent hypotheses that (a) family resilience in one's current family will be higher than in one's family of origin; (b) family resilience in one's family of origin and in one's current family will be negatively associated with alcohol abuse symptoms. The analysis, using SPSS software, proceeded in three steps. First, descriptive characteristics and bivariate relationships between the independent variables (e.g., family resilience – family of origin and family resilience – current family) and alcohol abuse symptoms were examined, following the conceptual model. Second, significant differences between family resilience in one's family of origin versus one's current family were determined using a paired sample t-test. Third, hierarchical regression was used to examine the multivariate main effects of the predictor variables. This analysis identified the specific amount of variance in alcohol abuse symptoms that was accounted for in three different steps (George & Mallery, 2013). In Step 1, demographic variables (gender, age, marital status, educational attainment, and income) were entered. In Step 2, perceptions of family resilience in one's family of origin were added. In Step 3, perceptions of family resilience in one's current family were added to the model. Listwise deletion was used for missing data. No multicollinearity problems were observed among all independent variables.

Measures

Demographics

Age (raw), gender (male/female), educational attainment (higher levels indicated by higher numbers), and marital status (single, engaged, living together, or married) were included in the models as controls. Annual household income at the ordinal level, ranging from 1 (*less than 2,000 USD*) to 9 (*greater than 100,000 USD*) was also reported (See Table 1).

Alcohol use

Individual's abuse symptoms were measured by the CAGE questionnaire, which stands for the extent a person thought they should Cut down, were Annoyed, Guilty, or had an Eye opener related to drinking (Ewing, 1984). Participants indicated yes/no (0/1), and when added, any score that is 2 or above is clinically significant. Cronbach's alpha was.88.

Family resilience – upbringing and current family

Family resilience was assessed through a 20-item scale of family protective factors, the Family Resilience Inventory (Burnette et al., 2019), which was created from emergent qualitative results with the sample population. Participants completed a family of origin and current family measure. Items were added with a yes/no format and included, "We express love and affection freely (hugs, kisses, saying 'I love you')," and "We stick with each other through thick and thin." The total score ranged from 0–20 for each scale with higher values indicating greater family resilience. Cronbach's alpha was .88.

Qualitative results

Both the Inland and the Coastal tribes emphasized "love" as the most important thing that holds families together. Along with sticking with each other and showing understanding through hard times, participants tended to describe verbal, physical, and frequent rituals of affection as components of the love they described. Results are presented separately for each tribe. First, both tribes clearly, explicitly identified "Love" as an important aspect of their families.

Inland tribe

Participants emphasized love for their family members as the essence of family resilience and strength. A woman stated that love was the most important thing in her current family, stating: 'Love. Love. Love. You got to love your children. Love your father. Love your son. Daughter. ... They need to learn that." A male participant emphasized the importance of, "structure, and a deep love of a parent to stay behind them – but allow them to make mistakes and help them to succeed." Similarly, another woman stated: "I think, just show them [children] love. ... I think that is- it really starts with the parents. ... show some comfort and support and love." Twin boys in a family interview commented on how love made their family resilient: "I'd say it's our love for each other ... I know that because no matter what, we still stick together no matter what."

Coastal tribe

Participants in the Coastal Tribe also referenced the importance of love explicitly. A woman interviewed asserted that "the love" was what held her family together. Another woman emphasized the importance of, "Respect. Love." A man interviewed explained, "[A] strong family to me would be have a lot of love for each other, getting along, and I think that's the part of it, is love each other." Many Coastal tribal members spoke about not having a lot of economic resources but being rich in love. A participant in a family interview stated, "We were not rich. We were poor, but we were rich in being together and as a loving family." A woman interviewed related, "My mom passed away ... We always said we were poor but loved ... She raised us to love each other and to stand by each other and support each other. ... We do that to this day."

Verbal affection

Verbal expressions of love were essential ingredients to what participants perceived as love. Using loving words and letting family members know you love them was crucial.

Inland tribe

Telling children they were loved was considered important at any age in the Inland Tribe. A female participant noted that what matters in families is, "I guess it's really love. Now that I know what love is – how you, we [she and her son] talk – how you treat, how we treat each other ... what I say to him. You know, things like that. Everything is positive." Relatedly, when asked about what's important for families, a woman in a focus group, stated:

> Communication is the main key. ... That's another way to express all your feelings amongst each other, um, and show an affection – ... show that there is love in the home.

A woman in another focus group stated, "The communication part, too … – my child is – he's gonna be 22, um, but I still give him a hug, and tell him I love him." When asked about what keeps families together, this same woman replied, "The glue? It's the communication and, you know, telling them you love them." When asked how she knew she was cared for, another woman answered, "'Cause they always tell me when I'll feel down, or something. They'll tell me that they love me, and they'll take us out to eat."

Coastal tribe

Verbal affection was echoed as a valued means of expressing love among family members in the Coastal Tribe. One woman responded that "Love for each other" was the glue that held her and her extended family together. She added, "We're bonded. Like my brothers, the last three – it's like they on the boat [work on a boat], but every day, I talk to them. The one after me, every night he calls me and tells me, 'Goodnight, I love you,' and my other brothers, the little ones, they call. We just close." Similarly, a daughter in the family, describing phone calls with her sister, described, "When we hang up on the phone, before we hang up, she says, 'I love you.' I say, 'I love you more,' sometimes she say, 'I love you most.'"

Physical affection

For both tribes, physical affection was an important means of showing love for family members. Participants across tribes described hugs, kisses, and other forms of physical touch between many different family members as key indicators of love within the family.

Inland tribe

The importance of showing physical affection to children in the family was frequently emphasized by the Inland Tribe. A female participant described family affection for her children : "We both hug and kiss our kids. It's weird. My dad never did it to us, but with my kids, he'll hug and hold them and kiss them. Maybe it's different when it's your grandkids."

Physical affection was also perceived as an important component of comfort and support, particularly from mothers, consistent with recent research (Sabey et al., 2018). One female participant explained that she knew her mother cared for her because her mother helped her when she was in need and displayed physical affection, stating "She, uh, provides me with, uh, like, when I'm sad or something she'll help me or when I just want a hug." Similarly, another woman stated, "My mom kind of had a sixth sense when I was feeling down." This participant went on to remark that there was daily hugging and statements of "I love you".

Coastal tribe

Physical affection from parents to children was also frequently described in the Coastal tribe, with an emphasis on female caregivers. A woman interviewed stated, "My mom was very demonstrative. Hugs, kissing and that kind of stuff." A male participant described his mom: "She was affectionate. She always showed us love. She always tried to show us." Displaying affection for one another physically was also important to maintain closeness amongst other family members. A woman from the Coastal Tribe described how her parents showed their affection, explaining, "Where one went, the other one went."

A mother in a family interview stated the glue that held the family together was, "That connection and love." When asked how she knows, she answered: "If I'm simply just watching TV … I may say go get a blanket and then we'll cuddle together. … I think once you get too busy for those little things you end up with distance." As her statement shows, those "little things" are considered important ways that families show love to one another regularly.

Frequent rituals of love and affection

Participants from both tribes emphasized the presence of loving rituals as a part of daily activities. Like many rituals, these interactions between family members are a part of the family routine, often occurring at specific times each day.

Inland tribe

For example, when asked how she knew she was cared for, a woman stated, "Our love, I think." This participant stated she knew she was loved, "Because every night, we will tell each other [they love each other] and everything before we go to bed." Another woman recalled her most positive memories growing up based on the love her parents showed through their daily routines, stating:

> "I had the best parents, I would say. Because they always participated in every school activity that parents were allowed to get in and stuff. They always told me they loved me a lot – Every time I'd go to sleep and everything. We still do. Yeah. Every time I go somewhere, I always give hug and kisses before I go and everything."

Coastal tribe

In the Coastal Tribe, rituals of love were frequently described as important parts of the family routine. One woman interviewed highlighted the importance of rituals of verbal and physical expressions of affection, explaining, "Yeah, before we'd go to bed, 'Good night, I love you.' Before we'd leave for school, 'Bye, I love you.' Always give a hug and a kiss on the cheek."

Participants in a family interview described a simple ritual of verbal affection between parents and children, and between siblings: "We hang up [the phone], we say to each other, 'We love you.' She say, 'We love you more.'"

Generational changes in expressions of love

Across both tribes, participants often described how the ways that they express love have changed from one generation to the next. The most common example of this was participants' statements revealing a contrast between the relative lack of open expression of love during their upbringing in their families of origin compared to the intentional and explicit expression of love practiced in their current families.

Inland tribe

While many members of the Inland Tribe express love and affection in their current families, a number of interviewees reported that they did not experience such open expressions of love during their upbringing. A woman explained that the lack of parental affection during her childhood resulted in parenting her own children differently, stating:

> I love my kids. We give each other hugs and tell each other we love each other and that kind of thing that my grandmother never used to do to us, or my mother never did to us. Everything that they never did to us, I do for them. I ... try to teach them things.

Echoing this, a man in a family interview expressed:

> My family ... they never gave us that love and affection. I don't think most Indians do that. They don't hug. ... I try to teach my kids different. ... . I want them to love each other and have respect for each other. ... I don't think too many families around here hug their kids. They never tell each other they love each other. I try to raise my kids different.

Similarly, a woman described the importance of love within the family, and indicated that the absence of open expressions of love amongst tribal members was cause for concern, stating:

"I think the [Tribal members] never say 'I love you' to the kids. And that's what they need. They need attention." Also commenting on generational changes in the expression of love, a woman conveyed that she expresses love and affection, although she did not receive it as a child:

> My mom and dad ... I don't think they'd ever told us, "I love you." ... For me, raising my children and stuff ... that was kind of a learned thing. It was, it was hard for me to be affectionate, um, and to tell them that, that I love them. But I make a point of doing it.

Coastal tribe

Changes in the expression of love from generation to generation were also observed by members of the Coastal Tribe, with an emphasis on the lack of affection expressed from fathers to sons. A man interviewed described how the absence of love and affection in his family of origin taught him to be different with his own children, as stated:

> I'm the parent who I always wanted as a kid. I'm that parent to my kids, as far as someone who shows emotion to my kids, um, kisses them, hugs them, reads to them, talks to them, knows what's going on. Uh, I'm that parent that I wanted as a kid, which I never had.

Another man interviewed wished he had heard more words of affection growing up, stating his longing: "Probably to hear my dad tell me. I mean, he's still around now, but for me to hear him tell me he loved me more probably ... I might have heard that being said about five times in my life." He added, "My mom said it all the time," but that he needed that from his dad. He went on to explain the intergenerational cycle of a lack of affection from father figures:

> My dad didn't always say it because my grandpa probably never said it to him. ... He wasn't always going to tell you that he loved you, but his actions showed that he did. I don't think action is enough. ... If you don't say it, how are they going to ever hear it?

Similarly, a woman interviewed revealed the contrast between her family upbringing and the way she parents: "They're not really affectionate people. I'm like that with my kids though, I'm really affectionate. I guess that's why I am because I grew up with not that much affection, you know? I changed that cycle a lot." These qualitative results indicate that love is perceived as a critical aspect of family strength and resilience by members of both the Inland Tribe and the Coastal Tribe. The focus now turns to investigating these themes quantitatively.

Quantitative results

Based on qualitative results, quantitative analyses aimed to reveal a potential link between family resilience (of which, love is a component) and alcohol abuse, a prevalent and well-documented risk factor amongst tribal members. Qualitative results illustrating the changes in the expression of love between generations were particularly influential in formulating two hypotheses: (a) family resilience in one's current family will be higher than in one's upbringing; (b) family resilience in one's upbringing and in one's current family will be negatively associated with alcohol abuse symptoms. Confirmation of these hypotheses could serve to bolster qualitative results surrounding changes in the expression of love as a component of family resilience from one generation to the next, and provide initial evidence indicating that family resilience is a family-level protective factor against alcohol abuse.

The average score for alcohol abuse symptoms among participants was 0.7 (SD = 1.29 range = 0–4). In total, 73.2% (n = 93) of participants reported no alcohol abuse symptoms, whereas 21.2% (n = 27) of participants reported alcohol abuse symptoms in the clinically significant range. At the bivariate level, each of the independent variables was significantly associated ($p < .01$) with the dependent variable of alcohol abuse symptoms, in the expected direction – which supports our hypotheses (Family Resilience – Upbringing, $r = -.272$ $p < .003$; and Family Resilience – Current, $r = -.223$ $p < .015$).

A paired samples t-test was conducted to compare significant differences in family resilience in one's upbringing versus in one's current family. As predicted, family resilience in one's upbringing ($M = 16.06$, $SD = 4.94$), on average, was reported at lower levels than in one's current family ($M = 18.03$, $SD = 3.22$) affirming the tentative hypothesis based on qualitative results that verbal and physical affection and love, along with other family resilience indicators, are higher for the current family than one's family of origin ($t = 4.387$, $df = 118$, $p. <000$).

Table 2. Summary of Hierarchical Regression Analysis for Variables Predicting Alcohol Abuse Symptoms for Native American Adults (n=127)

Variable	Model 1	Model 2	Model 3
Demographic Factors	β	β	β
Gender	-.095	-.134	-.157
Age	-.008	-.008	-.010
Monthly Household Income	.036	.019	.029
Highest Grade in School	.064	.058	.072
Marital Status	.-070	-.042	-.157
Family Resilience – Upbringing		-.052*	-.032
Family Resilience – Current Family			-.085*
F	.963	1.567	2.047
R^2	.046	.086	.126
F change	.963	4.423*	4.591*
R^2 change	.046	.040	.041

*$p < .05$. **$p < .05$. ***$p < .001$

Table 2 depicts the regression analysis. For Step 1, demographic variables explained 4.6% of the variance (R^2), though education, age, gender, income, and marital status were not significant across any of the models. Family of origin resilience (Family Resilience – Upbringing) factors explained an additional 4% of the variance for a total of 8.6% of the variance (R^2) accounted for in this step. In the final step, current family resilience explained 12.6% of the variance (R^2), an increase of 4.1% from step two. The change in Step 2 was significant ($R = .293$, $R^2 = .086$, $F(1,100) = 1.567$, $p < .038$), as well as in Step 3 ($R = .356$, $R^2 = .126$, $F(1, 99) = 2.047$, $p < .035$), supporting the hypothesis that higher levels of family resilience both in one's current family and in one's upbringing are negatively associated with alcohol abuse symptoms.

Discussion

Qualitative

This article prioritized participants' own words in qualitative results, and explicitly honored their language and descriptions of resilient, strong families (Burnette et.al., 2014; 2017). Qualitative results overwhelming supported the expressed importance of love, manifested amongst family members in several ways including verbal affection, physical affection, and rituals of affection, and the resilience of sticking together through hard times and combatting struggle with understanding and support. In both tribes, participants described acts of verbal and physical affection as important expressions of love between parents and children, as well as other family members. Rituals of love and affection were incorporated into daily family routines by members of both tribes, offering the opportunity for love to be expressed and felt regularly. Parents from both tribes also provided insight into how they are breaking intergenerational cycles by openly expressing their love for their family members, especially children, although this was not always a common practice in previous generations. In the Inland Tribe, a lack of parental affection was perceived to be a risk factor for children; in the Coastal Tribe, lack of affection was commonly experienced between fathers and sons.

Qualitative results also suggested that verbal and physical expressions of love within the tribal communities involved in this research may have a gendered component, with females being more verbally and physically expressive across both tribes. Verbal affection was strongly associated with mothers and female caretakers, as it was most often mothers who described their own use of verbal affection with children, and other participants most often mentioned receiving verbal affection from their mothers and grandmothers. This is an important finding amongst Indigenous communities that warrants further research, as studies have shown that father love significantly impacts social, emotional, and cognitive outcomes for children and young adults (Li & Meier, 2017). However, results also indicate that cultural (and potentially gendered) norms surrounding the expression of love are changing over time. The present generation emphasizes open expressions of love and affection, especially from parents to children, which was perceived to be a shift from previous generations. Many participants reported that they learned from their childhood experiences that were significantly lacking in parental affection, breaking this inter-generational cycle by choosing to do things differently within their current families; thus family resilience may enable transcendence despite experiences of oppression (Burnette, 2016).

Quantitative

Quantitative results also revealed interesting phenomena. First, clinically significant alcohol abuse was present among 21% of the sample, a striking number. Supporting the data from qualitative results, family resilience during one's upbringing was, in fact significantly lower than in one's current family, indicating a revitalization and resurgence of loving behaviors. This may indicate that the current generation is beginning to transcend the effects of historical oppression and express love to a greater degree. Importantly, the FRI, a culturally-specific and validated measure (Burnette et.al., 2019), was used to conceptualize and measure family resilience in this study, which included specific items from the qualitative methods employed, namely, "We express love and affection freely (hugs, kisses, saying 'I love you'); we laugh a lot; I feel it is stable, safe, and predictable; we are close knit; we come together during hard times, rather than going our separate ways; and, we stick with each other through thick and thin."

Quantitative analysis also revealed that family resilience had an effect on alcohol abuse in both models. Family resilience in one's upbringing significantly impacted alcohol abuse symptoms in the 2nd model, however, the significance of this effect was not maintained in the 3rd model in which family resilience in one's current family was included. These results indicate that family resilience in one's current family mediates the impact of family resilience during upbringing on alcohol abuse symptoms. This provides the promise of changing and improving intergenerational patterns, and that current family promotive processes, such as the expression of love, are highly important in relation to alcohol abuse outcomes. Despite other research examining risk factors for alcohol abuse, such as parental substance abuse, this is the first known study that examines the potential association between family resilience and alcohol abuse, a glaring and well-documented health disparity among Indigenous peoples.

Limitations

This study used mixed methodology as part of an in-depth, culturally-grounded, and community-based research project, exploring Indigenous peoples' perceptions of love, and finding several significant variables associated with alcohol abuse symptoms for men and women across two tribes, despite a relatively small sample size. The qualitative and quantitative results bolster one another, and support the FHORT. Importantly, this is the first study to examine love as it relates to alcohol abuse, however, as with all studies, there are limitations to this work that merit discussion. First, results from this convenience sample cannot be generalized beyond their context. Second, all variables were assessed via self-report measures. Additionally, some variables, such as gender, age, and educational status were not found to be significant. Given the diversity of Indigenous peoples, these results require further investigation across distinct contexts and with larger samples for a fuller understanding.

Implications and future research

Given the frequency with which love came up as a theme in participants' own words, it is striking that a literature search on love yielded no current research on families, nor any research related to love, family resilience, and alcohol abuse. It is unlikely that the importance of love is limited to this sample. More qualitative and quantitative research examining love specifically is warranted, not only to honor the conceptions meaningful to the specific research participants included in study samples, but to investigate promising directions to prevent and address persistent health disparities, such as alcohol and other drug abuse. The intentional bridging of the gap between the conceptualizations of important factors, like love, proposed by participants versus researchers is a needed approach to increase the relevance and applicability of research to the families and communities it endeavors to impact. The development of alcohol abuse prevention and intervention efforts that involve the entire family system, and focus on facilitating the expression of love as a component of family resilience are promising clinical implications.

Acknowledgments

The authors thank the dedicated work and participation of the tribes who contributed to this work.

Disclosure statement

No potential conflict of interest was reported by the authors.

Funding

This work was supported by the Fahs-Beck Fund for Research and Experimentation Faculty Grant Program [grant number #552745]; The Silberman Fund Faculty Grant Program [grant #552781]; the Newcomb College Institute Faculty Grant at Tulane University, University

Senate Committee on Research Grant Program at Tulane University, the Global South Research Grant through the New Orleans Center for the Gulf South at Tulane University, The Center for Public Service at Tulane University, and the Carol Lavin Bernick Research Grant at Tulane University. This work was supported, in part, by Award K12HD043451 from the Eunice Kennedy Shriver National Institute of Child Health & Human Development of the National Institutes of Health (Krousel-Wood-PI; Catherine McKinley (Formerly Burnette) Building Interdisciplinary Research Careers in Women's Health (BIRCWH) Scholar). Supported in part by U54 GM104940 from the National Institute of General Medical Sciences of the National Institutes of Health, which funds the Louisiana Clinical and Translational Science Center. The content is solely the responsibility of the authors and does not necessarily represent the official views of the National Institutes of Health.

ORCID

Catherine E. McKinley ⓘ http://orcid.org/0000-0002-1770-5088
Jenn Miller Scarnato ⓘ http://orcid.org/0000-0002-2485-943X

References

Armstrong, L. L., & Manion, I. G. (2015). Meaningful youth engagement as a protective factor for youth suicidal ideation. *Journal of Research on Adolescence*, *25*(1), 20–27. https://doi.org/10.1111/jora.12098

Barnert, E. S., Perry, R., Azzi, V. F., Shetgiri, R., Ryan, G., Dudovitz, R., Zima, B., & Chung, P. J. (2015). Incarcerated youths' perspectives on protective factors and risk factors for juvenile offending: A qualitative analysis. *American Journal of Public Health*, *105*(7), 1365–1371. https://doi.org/10.2105/AJPH.2014.302228

Bassuk, E, Dawson, R, & Huntington, N. (2006). Intimate partner violence in extremely poor women: longitudinal patterns and risk markers. *Journal Of Family Violence*, *21*(6), 387-399.

Bauer, M. S. (2016). Hope, faith, love, and treating serious mental health conditions. *American Journal of Psychiatry*, *173*(4), 319–320. https://doi.org/10.1176/appi.ajp.2016.15121604

Breton, J. J., Labelle, R., Berthiaume, C., Royer, C., St-Georges, M., Ricard, D., Guile, J. M., Cohen, D., Guilé, J.-M., & Abadie, P. (2015). Protective factors against depression and suicidal behaviour in adolescence. *Canadian Journal of Psychiatry.Revue Canadienne De Psychiatrie*, *60*(2 Suppl 1), S5–S15. https://www.ncbi.nlm.nih.gov/pmc/articles/PMC4345848/

Bureau of Indian Affairs. (2020). About us. Retrieved from https://www.bia.gov/about-us

Burnette, C. E. (2015). Historical oppression and intimate partner violence experienced by Indigenous women in the U.S.: understanding connections. *Social Services Review*, *89*(3), 531-563. http://www.jstor.org/stable/10.1086/683336

Burnette, C. E. (2016). Historical oppression and Indigenous families: uncovering potential risk factors for Indigenous families touched by violence. *Family Relations*, *65*(2), 354-368. doi: 10.1111/fare.12191

Burnette, C. E. (2017). Family and cultural protective factors as the bedrock of resilience for Indigenous women who have experienced violence. *Journal Of Family Social Work*, *21*(1), 45-62. doi: 10.1080/10522158.2017.1402532

Burnette, C. E. (2017). Family and cultural protective factors as the bedrock of resilience for Indigenous women who have experienced violence. *Journal Of Family Social Work*, *20*(5) doi: 10.1080/10522158.2017.1402532

Burnette, C. E., Boel-Studt, S., Renner, L. M., Figley, C. R., & Theall, K. P., *Miller Scarnato, J. & Billiot, S. (2019). The Family Resilience Inventory: A Culturally Grounded Measure of Intergenerational Family Protective Factors. (Early View/Advance online). Family Process, doi: doi:10.1111/famp.12423. PubMed PMCID:6716378

Burnette, C. E, & Figley, C. R. (2016). Risk and protective factors related to the wellness of American Indian and Alaska Native youth: a systematic review. *International Public Health Journal*, *8*(2), 137-154.

Burnette, C. E, & Figley, C. R. (2017). Historical oppression, resilience, and transcendence: Can a holistic framework help explain violence experienced by indigenous people? Social Work, *62*(1), 37-44.

Burnette, C. E, Sanders, S, Butcher, H. K, & Rand, J. T. (2014). A toolkit for ethical and culturally sensitive research: an application with Indigenous communities. *Ethics and Social Welfare*, *8*(4), 364-382. doi: 10.1080/17496535.2014.885987

Carspecken, P. (1996). *Critical ethnography in educational research, a theoretical and practical guide.* New York, NY: Routledge.

Chartier, K, & Caetano, R. (2010). Ethnicity and health disparities in alcohol research. *Alcohol Research & Health*, *33*(1–2), 152.

Creswell, J. W. (2015). *A concise introduction to mixed methods research.* Sage Publications.

Ewing, J. A. (1984). Detecting alcoholism: The CAGE questionnaire. *JAMA*, *252*(14), 1905–1907. https://doi.org/10.1001/jama.1984.03350140051025

George, D., & Mallery, P. (2013). *IBM SPSS statistics 21 step by step: A simple guide and reference.* Pearson.

Graham, J. M. (2011). Measuring love in romantic relationships: A meta-analysis. *Journal of Social and Personal Relationships*, *28*(6), 748–771. https://doi.org/10.1177/0265407510389126

Guest, G., & MacQueen, K. M. (2008). *Handbook for team-based qualitative research.* (G. Guest & K. M. MacQueen, Eds.). Altamira Press.

Gulledge, A. K., Hill, M., Lister, Z., & Sallion, C. (2007). Non-erotic physical affection: It's good for you. In L'Abate L. (Ed.), *Low-cost approaches to promote physical and mental health* (pp. 371–384). New York, NY: Springer.

Heshmati, S., Oravecz, Z., Pressman, S., Batchelder, W. H., Muth, C., & Vandekerckhove, J. (2017). What does it mean to feel loved: Cultural consensus and individual differences in felt love. *Journal of Social and Personal Relationships*, (Advance-online publication). https://doi.org/10.1177/0265407517724600.

Karandashev, V. (2015). A cultural perspective on romantic love. *Online Readings in Psychology and Culture*, *5*(4), 2. https://doi.org/10.9707/2307-0919.1135

LaFromboise, T. D., Hoyt, D. R., Oliver, L., & Whitbeck, L. B. (2006). Family, community, and school influences on resilience among American Indian adolescents in the upper Midwest. *Journal of Community Psychology*, *34*(2), 193–209. https://doi.org/10.1002/jcop.20090

León-del-Barco, B., Fajardo-Bullón, F., Mendo-Lázaro, S., Rasskin-Gutman, I., & Iglesias-Gallego, D. (2018). Impact of the familiar environment in 11–14-year-old minors' mental health. *International Journal of Environmental Research and Public Health*, *15*(7), 1314. https://doi.org/10.3390/ijerph15071314

Li, X., & Meier, J. (2017). Father love and mother love: Contributions of parental acceptance to children's psychological adjustment. *Journal of Family Theory & Review*, *9*(4), 459–490. https://doi.org/10.1111/jftr.12227

Lowe, S. R., Joshi, S., Pietrzak, R. H., Galea, S., & Cerdá, M. (2015). Mental health and general wellness in the aftermath of hurricane Ike. *Social Science & Medicine, 124*, 162–170. https://doi.org/10.1016/j.socscimed.2014.11.032

Martin, D., & Yurkovich, E. (2014). "Close-knit" defines a healthy Native American Indian family. *Journal of Family Nursing, 20*(1), 51–72. https://doi.org/10.1177/1074840713508604

Masten, A. S, & Monn, A. R. (2015). Child and family resilience: a call for integrated science, practice, and professional training. *Family Relations, 64*(1), 5-21.

McHugh, M. L. (2012). Interrater reliability: The kappa statistic. *Biochemia Medica, 22*(3), 276–282. https://doi.org/10.11613/BM.2012.031

Noller, P. (1996). What is this thing called love? Defining the love that supports marriage and family. *Personal Relationships, 3*(1), 97–115. https://doi.org/10.1111/j.1475-6811.1996.tb00106.x

Qualtrics, L. (2014). *Qualtrics [software]*. Qualtrics, Provo, UT, USA.

Riehl-Emde, A., Thomas, V., & Willi, J. (2003). Love: An important dimension in marital research and therapy. *Family Process, 42*(2), 253–267. https://doi.org/10.1111/j.1545-5300.2003.42205.x

Sabey, A. K., Rauer, A. J., Haselschwerdt, M. L., & Volling, B. (2018). Beyond "Lots of hugs and kisses": Expressions of parental love from parents and their young children in two-parent, financially stable families. *Family Process, 57*(3), 737–751. https://doi.org/10.1111/famp.12327

Sarche, M, & Spicer, P. (2008). Poverty and health disparities for American Indian and Alaska Native children: current knowledge and future prospects. *Annals Of The New York Academy Of Sciences, 1136*(), 126-136.

Schmitt, D. P., Youn, G., Bond, B., Brooks, S., Frye, H., Johnson, S., Sherrill, M., Sampias, J., Sherrill, M., Stoka, C., & Klesman, J. (2009). When will I feel love? The effects of culture, personality, and gender on the psychological tendency to love. *Journal of Research in Personality, 43*(5), 830–846. https://doi.org/10.1016/j.jrp.2009.05.008

Sternberg, R. J. (1986). A triangular theory of love. *Psychological Review, 93*(2), 119. https://doi.org/10.1037/0033-295X.93.2.119

Thayer, Z, Barbosa-Leiker, C, McDonell, M, Nelson, L, Buchwald, D, & Manson, S. (2017). Early life trauma, post-traumatic stress disorder, and allostatic load in a sample of American Indian adults. *American Journal of Human Biology, 29*(3), e22943.

Tolan, P, Gorman-Smith, D, & Henry, D. (2006). Family violence. *Annu. Rev. Psychol., 57*(), 557-583.

Walsh, F. (2016). Applying a family resilience framework in training, practice, and research: Mastering the art of the possible. *Family Process, 55*(4), 616–632. https://doi.org/10.1111/famp.12260

Whitbeck, L. B., Chen, X., Hoyt, D. R., & Adams, G. W. (2004). Discrimination, historical loss and enculturation: Culturally specific risk and resiliency factors for alcohol abuse among American Indians. *Journal of Studies on Alcohol, 65*(4), 409–418. https://doi.org/10.15288/jsa.2004.65.409

Xu, M. K., Morin, A. J., Marsh, H. W., Richards, M., & Jones, P. B. (2018). Psychometric validation of the parental bonding instrument in a UK population–based sample: Role of gender and association with mental health in mid-late life. *Assessment, 25*(6), 716–728. https://doi.org/10.1177/1073191116660813

Yu, M., & Stiffman, A. R. (2007). Culture and environment as predictors of alcohol abuse/dependence symptoms in American Indian youths. *Addictive Behaviors, 32*(10), 2253–2259. https://doi.org/10.1016/j.addbeh.2007.01.008

Diabetes, mental health, and utilization of mental health professionals among Native Hawaiian and Pacific Islander adults

Angela R. Fernandez ⓘ and Michael S. Spencer

ABSTRACT

National reports of diabetes and mental health for Native Hawaiian and Pacific Islanders (NHPI) are high, yet mental health professional access is low. We used multiple logistic regression to analyze data from the 2014 NHPI National Health Interview Survey. We evaluated the association between diabetes and serious psychological distress, and the interaction effect of mental health professional utilization among 2,587 adults. Self-reported diabetes was positively associated with serious psychological distress, but mental health professional utilization did not affect this association. Stigma and measurement gaps may influence self-report and measurement of mental health symptomatology, suggesting the need for culturally grounded approaches.

Introduction

Mental health symptomatology is common among people living with or at risk for diabetes (Centers for Disease Control and Prevention [CDC], 2018). Across communities of color, racial discrimination has been shown to add additional stressors that can potentially exacerbate mental health symptomatology among individuals with diabetes (LeBrón et al., 2019; LeBron et al., 2014; Spencer et al., 2006; Walls et al., 2014). For Native Hawaiian and Pacific Islanders (NHPI), race/ethnicity is a predictor for diabetes-related stress (Boden & Gala, 2018).

There are no national studies to date that examine the associations between diabetes, mental health symptomatology, and mental health professional utilization among NHPI populations. NHPI-specific national or local studies that evaluate whether mental health professional utilization buffers the relationship between diabetes status and mental health symptomatology is also lacking. In this study, we investigated the association between diabetes status and mental health symptomatology and examined mental health professional utilization as a potential interacting variable on this association.

Background

Approximately 1.2 million people living in the U.S. identify as NHPI alone or in combination with at least one other race, and represent about 0.4% of the nation's population (Hixson et al., 2012). The Federal Office of Management and Budget defines NHPI as people who culturally and ethnically descend from Hawaii, Samoa, Guam, and other Pacific Islands (Galinsky, Zelaya, Simile et al., 2017). NHPI are among the populations in the U.S. experiencing the most rapid population growth rate (Narcisse et al., 2018), and they also bear a markedly higher burden of chronic diseases compared with both Asian Americans and the U.S. population as a whole (Wu & Bakos, 2017). While the disaggregation of NHPI data from their previous categorization within the Asian American race has increased, NHPI continue to be underrepresented in health research (Narcisse et al., 2018).

Diabetes and mental health are among the top reported health diagnoses among NHPI nationally (Galinsky, Zelaya, Barnes et al., 2017). The 2014 NHPI National Health Information Survey (NHIS), the first national survey on NHPI, indicates that they are 2.4 times as likely to be diagnosed with diabetes compared with non-Hispanic whites (17.6% and 7.3%, respectively; Office of Minority Health, 2016). The national prevalence (adjusted for sex) of diabetes among NHPI adults is 15.6%, greater than both U.S. adults and single-race Asian adults. A total of 4.1% of NHPI (also adjusted for sex) also reported serious psychological distress in the past 30 days – greater than percentages among single-race Asian adults (Galinsky, Zelaya, Barnes et al., 2017). Earlier analysis of the national Behavioral Risk Factor Surveillance System revealed one-fifth of NHPI adults reported a depressive disorder diagnosis – a higher percentage than for all other U.S. racial groups. Anxiety disorder was reported as second highest (15.7%), just behind American Indians/Alaska Natives (Cook et al., 2010). Such disproportionate figures are concerning, given the evidence of co-morbidity between diabetes and mental health conditions among the U.S. population (CDC, 2018).

Within the U.S., people with diabetes are at two-three times greater risk of experiencing depression and 20% more likely to experience anxiety compared with people without diabetes, yet only one-quarter to one-half of people with diabetes are diagnosed and treated. Furthermore, one-third to one-half of people with diabetes experience diabetes distress, or feelings of discouragement, worry, frustration, or fatigue in daily diabetes care management (CDC, 2018). Racial/ethnic minorities may experience additional race-related stressors related to demographics, discrimination, daily hassles, or support of health care providers that can exacerbate diabetes-related distress and lead to mental health symptoms (LeBron et al., 2014; Spencer et al., 2006). One recent study of Latinos with diabetes found a positive association between racial/ethnic discrimination and depressive symptoms, and that such discrimination also mediated HbA1 c (blood glucose measured to help diagnose and monitor diabetes) levels through diabetes-related distress (LeBron et al., 2014). For NHPI individuals compared with white/ Caucasians, race/ethnicity also has a significant and positive association with diabetes-related stress (Boden & Gala, 2018).

The literature also points to the important role of culture in shaping and developing treatment approaches. For example, Latinos who received a culturally relevant, theory-based community health worker intervention experienced a significant decrease in diabetes-related distress. This suggests the potential effectiveness of culturally appropriate, community-based mental health care provision for other ethnic/racial minorities such as NHPI (Spencer et al., 2018). Furthermore, culturally based interventions are recognized as important when addressing overall NHPI health (Hurdle, 2002; Mokuau, 2011). These include culturally adapted diabetes interventions, which have shown promising results in addressing a range of health disparities (McElfish et al., 2019), as well as positive effects on improving diabetes self-management (Sinclair et al., 2013).

While no national-level, disaggregated survey data for NHPI with diabetes could be found regarding mental health diagnoses or utilization of mental health professionals, previous, more localized research illuminates the associations between diabetes and mental health symptomatology among NHPI. One study of a sample of Native Hawaiians in North Kohala, Hawaii, found a significant association between HbA1 c (at or above 7%) and depressive symptoms (adjusting for age, BMI, gender, and education, and excluding participants with a self-reported history of diabetes). The researchers did not find a statistically significant relationship between diabetes history and depressive symptoms (adjusting for HbA1c). They also adjusted for other confounders including age, BMI, gender, and education, concluding that the diabetes–depression association may be partially influenced by neuroendocrinological health issues (Grandinetti et al., 2000). There are also no studies to date that evaluate whether mental health professional utilization as a psychosocial variable could have an interacting effect on mental health symptomatology among those with diabetes. The strength of this association is hypothesized to vary as a function of such variables and may have "direct clinical implications for the treatment of depressive symptoms in people with diabetes" (Kaholokula et al., 2003, p. 439).

Both Native Hawaiian and non-Native Hawaiian psychologists have called for an increased study of Native Hawaiian mental health in response to the gap in empirical work on this issue. Particularly, they have highlighted the importance of ethnic identity and cultural practices in interventions

(Winerman, 2004). One potential challenge to both research and mental health care utilization among NHPI compared with the general U.S. public may lie in the higher levels of social stigma toward conceptions of mental health as a Westernized notion (Subica et al., 2019; Yamada et al., 2019). The Westernized notion is often considered incongruent with Indigenous conceptions of mental wellness. Grounded in holistic, interconnected principles of mind, body, and spirit connection, mental wellness is cultivated within family relationships and spiritual and land-based practices, since land is viewed as more than a physical location and as a source of physical, psychological, and spiritual nourishment essential to well-being (McCubbin & Marsella, 2009; Mokuau, 2011; Yamada et al., 2019). Thus, NHPI seek mental health support through family, spirituality, and cultural sources (McCubbin & Marsella, 2009; Yamada et al, 2019). Therefore, it is crucial for researchers and practitioners to understand the impacts of colonization and the resulting historical trauma on NHPI social determinants of health, as well as the potentially protective role of culture in addressing mental health issues within the NHPI community (McCubbin & Marsella, 2009; Subica et al., 2019).

Empirical studies based on national-level health data are emerging and can provide a source of data from which culturally appropriate studies can be drawn. The NHPI NHIS revealed important information about the current health status of the NHPI population across the nation. While health care access and utilization (Zelaya et al., 2017) and emergency department and outpatient service use have been analyzed from the NHPI NHIS (Narcisse et al., 2018), the association between diabetes and mental health symptomatology as well as the effects of mental health professional utilization have not yet been examined at the national level. In this study, we hypothesized a positive association between having diabetes and/or borderline/prediabetes and serious psychological distress. We also hypothesized that individuals with diabetes or borderline/prediabetes who had utilized mental health professional services would be less likely to score positively for serious psychological distress.

Methods

As the first-of-its-kind federal population-level study designed to evaluate the health of NHPI across the United States, the NHPI NHIS used the annual, cross-sectional NHIS as a survey instrument for data collection. The NHIS is a program of the National Center for Health Statistics (NCHS), which is part of the U.S. Centers for Disease Control and Prevention (CDC, 2017). As both the largest national household survey and the primary source of health information data in the U.S., it is used to collect data on health status and conditions, disability, risk factors, health service access and utilization, health insurance coverage, immunizations, and health-related behaviors. The NHPI NHIS resulted from a combination of progression on federal policies surrounding data collection guidelines and advocacy from Native Hawaiian, Pacific Islander, and Asian American health researchers, leaders, and community organizations, who recognized the need for disaggregation of NHPI from the single Asian and Pacific Islander racial and ethnic category in order to reduce the suppression of important health distinctions between groups (Wu & Bakos, 2017). Concurrently, to address the methodological challenges of including small sample populations such as NHPI in large-scale national surveys like the NHIS, the NCHS and Office of Minority Health used the American Community Survey as a sampling frame (Wu & Bakos, 2017). Stratified, multi-stage area probability sampling was used by the NCHS to ensure NHPI were properly represented among the larger U.S. population (Narcisse et al., 2018). For the NHPI NHIS, interviewers received cultural awareness, sensitivity and outreach training, and materials for communications with participants (i.e., advance notice and thank-you letters) were tailored to be culturally appropriate. Beyond these specific cultural adaptations designed to increase engagement with hard-to-reach, small populations such as NHPI, the NHPI NHIS followed all other standard protocols in order to ensure comparability of results with those of the standard NHIS (Narcisse et al., 2018).

The NHPI NHIS included a sample of approximately 3,000 households across all 50 states and the District of Columbia, in which at least one NHPI person resided during the year of 2014. The NHPI NHIS used an in-person survey with at least one household member of any age who self-reported as NHPI, whether alone or in combination with at least one other race (Wu & Bakos, 2017). NHPI were randomly selected from within these households to respond to the NHPI NHIS (Galinsky, Zelaya, Barnes et al., 2017). A more detailed description of the parent survey design methodology can be found in the NCHS Survey Description publication (CDC, 2017). This study involved secondary data analysis from the 2014 NHPI NHIS. It focused on a subsample (n = 2,587) of the total number of adults surveyed (n = 2,590). Subsample participants identified NHPI as their primary race (whether NHPI alone or in combination with one or more other races), and self-reported having a diabetes diagnosis (n = 381), borderline/prediabetes (n = 95), or reported not having diabetes or borderline/prediabetes (n = 2,111).

Measures

Serious psychological distress was our dependent variable, with a composite of six questions asking the frequency with which respondents felt "sad," "nervous," "restless or fidgety," that "everything was an effort," or "worthless during the past 30 days." Response options were displayed on a Likert scale (1 = all of the time, 5 = none of the time; CDC, 2017), and were coded from 0–4 for a total range of 0–24 on the serious psychological distress scale (A. M. Galinsky, Zelaya, Barnes et al., 2017). A score of 13 or higher categorized participants as experiencing serious psychological distress (Kessler, 2003; Kessler et al., 2003). *Diabetes status*, the predictor variable, required respondents to self-report "yes," "no," or "borderline or prediabetes" in response to whether they had been told by a doctor or other health care professional that they have "diabetes or sugar diabetes," (CDC, 2017). We examined all three categories as predictors (Galinsky, Zelaya, Simile et al., 2017). Finally, *having seen or spoken to a mental health professional in the past year* was the interacting variable and required a "yes" or "no" response (Baron & Kenny, 1986; CDC, 2017). Mental health professionals listed included a psychiatrist, psychologist, psychiatric nurse, or clinical social worker.

We also controlled for several covariates. *Sex* was predetermined as "male" or "female," and we recoded it from 1 and 2 to 0 and 1, respectively. *Age* was originally continuous, and we recoded it to be dichotomous ("54 and below" = 0; "55 and above" = 1). *Level of education completed* was recoded into dichotomous categories ("high school/GED and below" = 0; "some college and above" = 1). Finally, *marital status* was recoded into dichotomous categories ("not partnered" = 0; ("partnered" = 1).

Analyses

We used R for statistical analyses (R Core Team, 2019). We recoded all "refused," (n = 1) "not ascertained," (n = 0) and "don't know" (n = 2) responses to variable questions as missing data that were not included in the analysis, resulting in the aforementioned subsample of 2,587. For our descriptive analysis, we calculated percentages for categorical variables. For our inferential analysis, we used multivariate logistic regression to investigate the association between diabetes and serious psychological distress outcomes, as well as to examine mental health professional utilization as an interacting variable on this association. We used a chi-square to test the association among all covariates and the outcome variable in order to determine independence and use in our model. In Model 1, we regressed sex, age, educational level, and partnership status on serious psychological distress. In Model 2, we regressed no diabetes and borderline/prediabetes (diabetes as reference category) on serious psychological distress, controlling for all of the aforementioned covariates. In Model 3, we removed the diabetes variables and added having utilized mental health professional services to all of the same covariates regressed on serious psychological distress. In Model 4, we brought no diabetes and borderline/prediabetes (diabetes as reference group) back in as independent variables, controlling for all other aforementioned covariates. In Model 5, we added an interaction term (Baron & Kenny, 1986) between no diabetes and borderline/prediabetes (diabetes as reference group) and controlled for all aforementioned covariates. To examine the association between the dichotomous (i.e., no diabetes vs diabetes combined with borderline/prediabetes) and trichotomous versions of the diabetes variables across the models, we also used a likelihood ratio test and found no significant difference ($P = .23$). This finding supported our choice of using the trichotomous version of the diabetes variable to capture important qualitative differences between being borderline/prediabetic and having diabetes. We reported results of our inferential analysis using 95% confidence intervals and $\alpha = 0.05$ as our threshold for statistical significance.

Results

Table 1 displays the results of the descriptive analysis. The majority of respondents (81%) reported no diabetes, 15% reported diabetes, and 4% reported borderline/prediabetes. By sex, respondents who reported no diabetes and those who reported diabetes were nearly split in half, while those that reported borderline/prediabetes were slightly more likely to be female (58%). Regarding educational status, those reporting positive diabetes and borderline/prediabetes diagnoses were nearly split in half, while those not

Table 1. Demographic characteristics of Native Hawaiian and Pacific Islanders living in the U.S. by diabetic status from the 2014 national health interview survey.

Participant characteristics	Diabetes status (N = 2587[a])		
	Yes	No	Borderline/prediabetes
Total by diabetes status	381 (15%)	2111 (81%)	95 (4%)
Sex			
Male	193 (51%)	997 (47%)	40 (42%)
Female	188 (49%)	1114 (53%)	55 (58%)
Age			
18–54	132 (35%)	1521 (72%)	50 (53%)
55+	249 (65%)	590 (28%)	45 (47%)
Educational status			
High school/GED & below	195 (52%)	866 (41%)	44 (46%)
Some college & above	183 (48%)	1240 (59%)	51 (54%)
Partnership status			
Not partnered	109 (29%)	745 (36%)	41 (44%)
Partnered	264 (71%)	1349 (64%)	53 (56%)
Serious psychological distress			
Yes	25 (7%)	77 (4%)	6 (6%)
No	342 (93%)	1975 (96%)	87 (94%)
Saw mental health professional			
Yes	26 (7%)	159 (8%)	14 (15%)
No	351 (93%)	1935 (92%)	81 (85%)

[a]One person responded "refused" and two people responded "don't know" to the diabetes status questions. These individuals were coded as missing and were not counted in the analysis.

reporting diabetes tended to have somewhat higher educational levels (59%). Overall, those who had partners tended to have higher percentages of diabetes (71%) and borderline/prediabetes (56%) than those who were not partnered. The largest discrepancies occurred among the mental health variables. Only 7% of diabetes, 6% of borderline/prediabetes, and 4% of no diabetes respondents scored positively for serious psychological distress. Furthermore, 7% of diabetes, 8% of no diabetes, and 15% of borderline/prediabetes respondents had utilized a mental health professional in the past year. The relationship between diabetes status and having utilized a mental health professional was statistically significant (P – value = 0.03) using a Chi-square test.

Table 2 shows the results of the multiple logistic regressions. We exponentiated our coefficients for greater ease in interpretation. The first model included age, sex, partnership status, and educational status. Having a partner and at least some college experience and higher, predicted less serious psychological distress. Model 2 added the diabetes measures. Not having a diabetes diagnosis, having a partner, and having at least some college experience and higher, predicted less serious psychological distress. Model 3 excluded diabetes measures and included the mental health professional measure. Not seeing a mental health professional, having

Table 2. Predictors of serious psychological distress among diabetic Native Hawaiian and Pacific Islanders living in the U.S. Who saw or talked to mental health professional in the past 12 months from the 2014 national health interview survey.

Participant characteristics	Model 1 OR (95% CI)	Model 2 OR (95% CI)	Model 3 OR (95% CI)	Model 4 OR (95% CI)	Model 5 OR (95% CI)
No diabetes		0.5*** (0.3, 0.7)		0.5*** (0.3, 0.8)	0.7 (0.3, 1.7)
Borderline/prediabetes		0.9 (0.4, 1.9)		0.5 (0.2, 1.3)	0.8 (0.2, 2.7)
Ages 55+	1.1 (0.8, 1.5)	1.1 (0.8, 1.5)	1.0 (0.7, 1.4)	1.0 (0.7, 1.4)	1.0 (0.7, 1.4)
Female sex	0.9 (0.6, 1.3)	0.8 (0.5, 1.1)	0.9 (0.6, 1.3)	0.8 (0.5, 1.1)	0.8 (0.5, 1.1)
Partnered	0.6*** (0.4, 0.8)	0.5*** (0.4, 0.8)	0.6** (0.5, 0.9)	0.6** (0.4, 0.9)	0.6** (0.4, 0.9)
Some college +	0.5*** (0.4, 0.7)	0.5*** (0.4, 0.7)	0.5*** (0.3, 0.7)	0.5*** (0.4, 0.7)	0.5*** (0.4, 0.7)
No mental health professional			0.1*** (0.1, 0.1)	0.1*** (0.1, 0.1)	0.2*** (0.1, 0.4)
No diabetes, no mental health professional					0.6 (0.2, 1.5)
Borderline/prediabetes, no mental health professional					0.6 (0.1, 3.5)
Intercept	0.1*** (0.1, 0.1)	0.2*** (0.1, 0.3)	0.5** (0.3, 0.8)	1.0 (0.6, 1.9)	0.7 (0.3, 1.7)

p < 0.1 **p < 0.05 ***p < 0.01
OR = odds ratio; CI = confidence interval.

a partner, and having at least some college experience or higher, predicted less serious psychological distress. Model 4 included all previously mentioned terms. Those who did not have diabetes were half as likely to experience serious psychological distress compared to those who did, adjusting for all other covariates. Model 5 added the interaction between having seen a mental health professional and the diabetes measures. While our previous Chi-square tests revealed statistical significance for both the diabetes and the mental health therapist variables, adding the mental health therapist variable as an interaction effect on diabetes rendered the previous statistically significant association no longer significant.

Discussion

The results of the descriptive analyses reveal that demographics of diabetes status by age, sex, and educational levels were similar to national estimates (CDC, 2020). While there is limited national data on partnership status among people with diabetes, existing data suggest that having a partner positively influences diabetes management, which could have implications for partnership as a protective factor for the two-thirds of partnered adults with diabetes in this sample (Haines et al., 2018). The most significant discrepancies lie in the low proportion of adults across all diabetes status categories who report serious psychological distress and who report having seen a mental health professional. Low usage of mental health treatment in this sample is comparable to national estimates (CDC, 2018). However, low reporting of serious psychological distress in this sample stands in contrast to higher reports of mental health symptomatology among NHPI (Cook et al., 2010) and national samples of the general population (CDC, 2018) may raise questions about culturally appropriate mental health measurement tools and access to care.

Our inferential analyses provided a more in-depth understanding of these data through use of multiple logistic regressions. Across all five models, partnership and higher educational status, as indicators of socioeconomic status, were consistently associated with lower odds of experiencing serious psychological distress. These findings are consistent with national data (CDC, 2020), and could implicate the potentially protective role that such socioeconomic factors could play as determinants of prevention (Uchima et al., 2019). Furthermore, adding the mental health professional variable to Models 3–5, revealed the positive association between seeing a mental health professional and reporting serious psychological distress. Overall, these findings may point to education levels, partnership status, and health care access as potential social determinants of health that can influence both self-report and prevalence of health outcomes (Blue Bird Jernigan et al., 2018; Liu & Alameda, 2011).

Ultimately, the focal point of our inferential analysis explored two hypotheses: (1) whether there was an association between having a diabetes diagnosis and serious psychological distress, and (2) that having seen or talked to a mental health professional would have an interacting effect on this association. Consonant with our first hypothesis that diabetes status would be associated with serious psychological distress controlling for age, sex, marital status, and education status, people with diabetes were indeed more likely to report serious psychological distress (Model 4). These findings are reflected in national data on diabetes and the increased likelihood of experiencing depression, anxiety, or diabetes distress (CDC, 2018). They were also reflected in American Indian data that showed a positive association between mental health symptoms and hyperglycemia (Walls et al., 2014) as well as localized data among Native Hawaiians that showed that high HbA1 c levels were associated with depressive symptoms (Grandinetti et al., 2000). Furthermore, while having seen a mental health professional was not a predictor of interest for Model 4, its statistical significance reveals that those who did see a mental health professional were around 10% more likely to have greater serious psychological distress. These results are also supported by a recent study (which included NHPI in its sample) that found that heightened diabetes-related stress was significantly and positively associated with seeking and/or receiving mental health treatment (Boden & Gala, 2018).

However, our second hypothesis – that having seen a mental health professional would influence the association between diabetes status and serious psychological distress – did not have a statistically significant impact on a respondent's likelihood of scoring positive for serious psychological distress (Model 5). While Model 5 did show that those who did not report a diabetes or borderline/prediabetes diagnosis were around 40% less likely to score positively for serious psychological distress than those who had these diagnoses and did see a mental health professional, these associations were not statistically significant. However, these findings could suggest another possible interpretation. First, given high levels of social stigma associated with mental health conditions (Subica et al., 2019; Yamada et al., 2019), self-report of mental health symptomatology may be less likely among NHPI. Within the NHIS, the NHPI study is the largest and only existing national health dataset of its kind, yet those respondents who had seen a mental health professional comprised just a fraction of the sample – from 7% to 15% across those who did and did not have diabetes or borderline/prediabetes. National data among the general population similarly reveals that while mental health treatment is typically effective in reducing symptomatology, the use of mental health treatment services among people with diabetes is nationally low (between one-quarter and one-half; CDC, 2018). Also, there is a shortage of mental health professionals in NHPI communities (Look et al., 2013; Yamada et al., 2019), and especially those who are perceived as linguistically and culturally responsive (Yamada et al., 2019). Second, the Westernized nature of the serious psychological distress measure may be incongruent with NHPI cultural conceptions of mental wellness (McCubbin & Marsella, 2009). This is possibly reflected in the 4% (no diabetes), 6% (borderline/prediabetes), and 7% (diabetes) response rates of the sample that scored positively on having symptoms of serious psychological distress. Third, NHPI may also seek out other informal sources of mental health support through spirituality and religion and family relationships (Yamada et al., 2019), as well as a range of traditional healing practices (McCubbin & Marsella, 2009), yet these variables are often excluded from research studies. Thus, mental health stigma, potential cultural deficits in the serious psychological distress measure, and the exclusion of variables that account for non-Western-centric mental health supports, together with the small subsample of those who responded positively to the independent, dependent, and potentially interacting variables, could help explain the lack of significant results.

Limitations

There were several limitations inherent in this data set. Its cross-sectional design prohibited the possibility of investigating the temporal relationship between diabetes as an exposure and serious psychological distress as an outcome. Furthermore, its reliance on self-reported data could have introduced selection bias and information bias of study variables. Also, there were no additional questions in the dataset that assessed other causes of psychological distress (e.g., other recent trauma in the past 30 days) and that could have been adjusted for. Furthermore, the NHPI NHIS, as a publicly available dataset, excludes geographical details such as zip codes, state of residence, or urban/rural setting, eliminating the possibility of considering settings-based health care distinctions by community and reducing potentially important variables for which to adjust (Narcisse et al., 2018).

Additionally, the small number of respondents who corresponded positively to the independent, dependent, and interacting variables gave limited statistical power to the estimation of the interaction, which thereby limited the model's ability to capture potential effects of the interaction. Consequently, the ternary nature of the interaction coupled with the scarcity of observations made the interaction somewhat imprecise. Consequently, the highly statistically significant ($P < .00$) association between having seen a mental health professional and the serious psychological distress outcome variable could have further contributed to the interaction term's lack of statistical significance (Boden & Gala, 2018). These factors combined with potential measurement error based on the aforementioned mental health stigma and lack of culturally relevant measurement tools (McCubbin &

Marsella, 2019; Subica et al., 2019), could have contributed to the lack of statistical significance for our hypothesized interaction.

Future studies could collect both cross-sectional and longitudinal data from a larger sample of people with diabetes and serious psychological distress. Culturally relevant measures of mental wellness could be developed by engaging community members in construct building through use of community-based participatory research approaches (McCubbin & Marsella, 2009; Panapasa et al., 2012) as well as including culturally grounded help-seeking variables such as use of traditional healing practices (Subica et al., 2019; Yamada et al., 2019) in mental health research. Such approaches would respond to NHPI scholars' and clinicians' calls for more research to examine these relationships (Kaholokula et al., 2003; Winerman, 2004) as an initial step toward building this body of literature.

Implications for practice

This study provides an initial glimpse into the mental health symptomatology and treatment of NHPI with diabetes or borderline/prediabetes. It is the first to provide national estimates of associations between diabetes and mental health conditions as comorbid health conditions, as well as estimates of mental health care utilization by NHPIs. Researchers, policy makers, and practitioners should focus their efforts on ensuring that mental health care services for NHPI with diabetes are culturally grounded and relevant to the NHPI population. This could increase the odds of mental health care utilization and effective treatment for this population. By conducting exploratory research that examines the discourse surrounding mental health and well-being within the NHPI community, we can further understand cultural perspectives surrounding wellness. This could help reduce stigma that may impede access to and quality of care, and further support culturally relevant measurement development. Accordingly, assessing availability of and access to culturally appropriate treatment could be crucial in building the necessary infrastructure to improve mental health outcomes among NHPI with diabetes or borderline/prediabetes.

Acknowledgments

With gratitude to Dr. Ann Downer for her editorial assistance.

Disclosure statement

The authors reported no potential conflict of interest.

Funding

This work was supported by the National Institute of General Medical Sciences of the National Institutes of Health under Award Number S06GM127164.

ORCID

Angela R. Fernandez ⬤ http://orcid.org/0000-0001-9066-7367

References

Baron, R., & Kenny, D. (1986). The moderator-mediator variable distinction in social psychological research: Conceptual, strategic, and statistical considerations. *Journal of Personality and Social Psychology, 51*(6), 1173–1182. https://doi.org/10.1037/0022-3514. 51.6.1173

Blue Bird Jernigan, V., D'Amico, E. J., Duran, B., & Buchwald, D. (2018). Multilevel and community-level interventions with Native Americans: Challenges and opportunities. *Prevention Science, 21*(Suppl 1), S65–S73. https://doi.org/10.1007/s11121-018-0916-3

Boden, M. T., & Gala, S. (2018). Exploring correlates of diabetes-related stress among adults with Type 1 diabetes in the T1D exchange clinic registry. *Diabetes Research and Clinical Practice, 138*, 211–219. https://doi.org/10.1016/j.diabres.2017.10.012

Centers for Disease Control and Prevention. (2017). *Native Hawaiian and Pacific Islander (NHPI) National Health Interview Survey (NHIS)*. U.S. Department of Health and Human Services. https://www.cdc.gov/nchs/nhis/nhpi.html

Centers for Disease Control and Prevention. (2020). *National diabetes statistics report, 2020*. U.S. Department of Health and Human Services. https://www.cdc.gov/diabetes/pdfs/data/statistics/national-diabetes-statistics-report.pdf

Centers for Disease Control Prevention. (2018). *Diabetes & mental health*. U.S. Department of Health and Human Services. https://www.cdc.gov/diabetes/managing/mental-health.html

Cook, W. K., Chung, C., & Ve'e, T. (2010). *Native Hawaiian and Pacific Islander health disparities*. Asian & Pacific Islander American Health Forum. https://www.apiahf.org/resource/native-hawaiian-and-pacific-islander-health-disparities/

Galinsky, A. M., Zelaya, C. E., Barnes, P. M., & Simile, C. (2017, March). *Selected health conditions among Native Hawaiian and Pacific Islander adults: United States, 2014* (NCHS Data Brief, (277)). U.S. Department of Health and Human Services. https://www.cdc.gov/nchs/data/databriefs/db277.pdf

Galinsky, A. M., Zelaya, C. E., Simile, C., & Barnes, P. M. (2017). Health conditions and behaviors of Native Hawaiian and Pacific Islander persons in the United States, 2014. *National Center for Health Statistics: Vital Health Statistics, 3*(40). U.S. Department of Health and Human Services. https://www.cdc.gov/nchs/data/series/sr_03/sr03_040.pdf

Grandinetti, A., Kaholokula, J. K., Crabbe, K. M., Kenui, C. K., Chen, R., & Chang, H. K. (2000). Relationship between depressive symptoms and diabetes among Native Hawaiians. *Psychoneuroendocrinology, 25*(3), 239–246. https://doi.org/10.1016/S0306-4530(99)00047-5

Haines, L., Coppa, N., Harris, Y., Wisnivesky, J. P., & Lin, J. J. (2018). The impact of partnership status on diabetes control and self-management behaviors. *Health Education & Behavior, 45*(5), 668–671. https://doi.org/10.1177/1090198117752783

Hixson, L. K., Hepler, B. B., & Kim, M. O. (2012, May). *The Native Hawaiian and Other Pacific Islander population: 2010.* U.S. Census Bureau. https://www.census.gov/prod/cen2010/briefs/c2010br-12.pdf

Hurdle, D. (2002). Native Hawaiian traditional healing: Culturally based interventions for social work practice. *Social Work, 47*(2), 183–192. https://doi.org/10.1093/sw/47.2.183

Kaholokula, J., Haynes, K., Grandinetti, S., & Chang, N. (2003). Biological, psychosocial, and sociodemographic variables associated with depressive symptoms in persons with type 2 diabetes. *Journal of Behavioral Medicine, 26*(5), 435–458. https://doi.org/10.1023/A:1025772001665

Kessler, R. (2003). *K6+ self-report measure.* [Measurement instrument]. World Health Organization. https://www.hcp.med.harvard.edu/ncs/ftpdir/k6/Self%20admin_K6.pdf

Kessler, R. C., Barker, P. R., Colpe, L. J., Epstein, J. F., Gfroerer, J. C., Hiripi, E., Howes, M. J., Normand, S.-L., Manderscheid, R. W., Walters, E. E., & Zaslavsky, A. M. (2003). Screening for serious mental illness in the general population. *Archives of General Psychiatry, 60*(2), 184–189. https://doi.org/10.1001/archpsyc.60.2.184

LeBrón, A., Spencer, M., Kieffer, W., Sinco, M., & Palmisano, E. (2019). Racial/ethnic discrimination and diabetes-related outcomes among Latinos with type 2 diabetes. *Journal of Immigrant and Minority Health, 21*(1), 105–114. https://doi.org/10.1007/s10903-018-0710-0

LeBron, A., Valerio, M., Kieffer, E., Sinco, B., Rosland, A., Hawkins, J., Espitia, N., Palmisano, G., & Spencer, M. (2014). Everyday discrimination, diabetes-related distress, and depressive symptoms among African Americans and Latinos with diabetes. *Journal of Immigrant and Minority Health, 16*(6), 1208–1216. https://doi.org/10.1007/s10903-013-9843-3

Liu, D. M., & Alameda, C. K. (2011). Social determinants of health for Native Hawaiian children and adolescents. *Hawaii Medical Journal, 70*(11: Suppl. 2), 9–14. https://pubmed.ncbi.nlm.nih.gov/22235151/

Look, M. A., Trask-Batti, M. K., Agres, R., Mau, M. L., & Kaholokula, J. K. (2013). *Assessment and priorities for health & well-being in Native Hawaiians & other Pacific Peoples.* Center for Native and Pacific Health Disparities Research. http://blog.hawaii.edu/uhmednow/files/2013/09/AP-Hlth-REPORT-2013.pdf

McCubbin, L., & Marsella, A. (2009). Native Hawaiians and psychology: The cultural and historical context of Indigenous ways of knowing. *Cultural Diversity and Ethnic Minority Psychology, 15*(4), 374–387. https://doi.org/10.1037/a0016774

McElfish, P., Purvis, A., Esquivel, R., Sinclair, S., Townsend, M., Hawley, K., Haggard-Duff, L. K., & Kaholokula, J. K. (2019). Diabetes disparities and promising interventions to address diabetes in Native Hawaiian and Pacific Islander populations. *Current Diabetes Reports, 19*(5), 1–9. https://doi.org/10.1007/s11892-019-1138-1

Mokuau, N. (2011). Culturally based solutions to preserve the health of Native Hawaiians. *Journal of Ethnic & Cultural Diversity in Social Work, 20*(2), 98–113. https://doi.org/10.1080/15313204.2011.570119

Narcisse, M., Felix, H., Long, C. R., Hudson, T., Payakachat, N., Bursac, Z., & McElfish, P. A. (2018). Frequency and predictors of health services use by Native Hawaiians and Pacific Islanders: Evidence from the U.S. National Health Interview Survey. *BMC Health Services Research, 18*(1), 1–14. https://doi.org/10.1186/s12913-017-2770-6

Office of Minority Health. (2016). *Diabetes and Native Hawaiians/Pacific Islanders.* U.S. Department of Health and Human Services. https://minorityhealth.hhs.gov/omh/browse.aspx?lvl=4&lvlid=78

Panapasa, S., Jackson, J., Caldwell, C., Heeringa, S., Mcnally, J., Williams, D., Coral, D., Taumoepeau, L., Young, L., Young, S., & Fa'asisila, S. (2012). Community-based participatory research approach to evidence-based research: Lessons from the Pacific Islander American health study. *Progress in Community Health Partnerships*, 6(1), 53–58. https://doi.org/10.1353/cpr.2012.0013

R Core Team. (2019). *R: A language and environment for statistical computing* [Computer software]. R Foundation for Statistical Computing. https://www.R-project.org/

Sinclair, K. A., Sinclair, E., Makahi, C., Shea-Solatorio, S., Yoshimura, C., Townsend, J., & Kaholokula, J. K. (2013). Outcomes from a diabetes self-management intervention for Native Hawaiians and Pacific People: Partners in care. *Annals of Behavioral Medicine: A Publication of the Society of Behavioral Medicine*, 45(1), 24–32. https://doi.org/10.1007/s12160-012-9422-1

Spencer, M., Kieffer, E., Sinco, B., Palmisano, G., Guzman, J., James, S., Graddy-Dansby, G., Two Feathers, J., & Heisler, M. (2006). Diabetes-specific emotional distress among African Americans and Hispanics with type 2 diabetes. *Journal of Health Care for the Poor and Underserved*, 17(2), 88–105. https://doi.org/10.1353/hpu.2006.0095

Spencer, M., Kieffer, E., Sinco, B., Piatt, G., Palmisano, G., Hawkins, J., LeBron, A., Espitia, N., Tang, T., Funnell, M., & Heisler, M. (2018). Outcomes at 18 months from a community health worker and peer leader diabetes self-management program for Latino adults. *Diabetes Care*, 41(7), 1414–1422. https://doi.org/10.2337/dc17-0978

Subica, A. M., Aitaoto, N., Sullivan, J. G., Henwood, B. F., Yamada, A. M., & Link, B. G. (2019, March). Mental illness stigma among Pacific Islanders. *Psychiatry Research*, 273, 578–585. https://doi.org/10.1016/j.psychres.2019.01.077

Uchima, O., Wu, Y. Y., Browne, C., & Braun, K. L. (2019). Disparities in diabetes prevalence among Native Hawaiians/Other Pacific Islanders and Asians in Hawai'i. *Preventing Chronic Disease*, 16(E22), 1–13. https://doi.org/10.5888/pcd16.180187

Walls, M., Aronson, B., Soper, G., & Johnson-Jennings, M. (2014). The prevalence and correlates of mental and emotional health among American Indian adults with type 2 diabetes. *The Diabetes Educator*, 40(3), 319–328. https://doi.org/10.1177/0145721714524282

Winerman, L. (2004, October). Psychologists call for increased study of Native Hawaiian mental health. *Monitor on Psychology*, 35(9), 20. https://www.apa.org/monitor/oct04/mentalhealth

Wu, S., & Bakos, A. (2017). The Native Hawaiian and Pacific Islander national health interview survey: Data collection in small populations. *Public Health Reports*, 132(6), 606–608. https://doi.org/10.1177/0033354917729181

Yamada, A., Vaivao, D., & Subica, A. (2019). Addressing mental health challenges of Samoan Americans in Southern California: Perspectives of Samoan community providers. *Asian American Journal of Psychology*, 10(3), 227–238. https://doi.org/10.1037/aap0000140

Zelaya, C. E., Galinsky, A. M., Simile, C., & Barnes, P. M. (2017). Health care access and utilization among Native Hawaiian and Pacific Islander persons in the United States, 2014. *National Center for Health Statistics: Vital Health Statistics*, 3(41) 1–79. https://www.ncbi.nlm.nih.gov/pubmed/30248011

Salud, cultura, tradición: Findings from an alcohol and other drug and HIV needs assessment in urban "Mexican American Indian" communities

Ramona Beltrán, Antonia R. G. Alvarez, Angela R. Fernandez ⓘ, Xochilt Alamillo, and Lisa Colón

ABSTRACT

This paper presents findings from an alcohol and other drug use (AOD) and HIV risk needs assessment of 20 "Mexican American Indian" adults in two urban areas of the United States who currently or previously participated in Danza Mexica an Indigenous cultural/ceremonial dance form. Findings describe community perceptions of AOD and HIV knowledge, stigma, and risk. The majority of participants identified AOD and more than half perceived HIV to be significant health concerns. Importantly, the majority of the participants also described specific teachings and practices from Danza Mexica related to AOD and HIV prevention and response, emphasizing cultural identity, community support, and healing.

Introduction

Changes to tribal groupings since the 2000 U.S. Census have revealed more diversity amongst those Indigenous peoples previously identified broadly as "Latin American Indians" (Norris et al., 2012). A 2012 U.S. Census Brief documents "Mexican American Indians" (MAI)[1] as the fourth largest tribal grouping in the U.S. (Norris et al., 2012). This raises important empirical questions about the population related to identity and identification associated with intersecting racial/ethnic and cultural identities as both Mexican and American Indian. Additionally, the complex confluence of previous and current migration experiences as well as histories of colonization, displacement, and persistent discrimination – factors associated with historical trauma – among the members of this community, point to questions about unique health risk and protective factors. As MAI serves as a blanket term for all people who have tribal affiliation or attachments to Indigenous groups of Mexico, there are likely subgroups within this broad tribal grouping category that are organized both around cultural identity and experience.

One of these groups is a community unified by traditional Indigenous cultural practices originating from Mexico, but centered on Danza Mexica (Aztec Dance), a cultural and ceremonial dance form practiced widely across North America and increasingly globally. Multiple components of the impacts of historical trauma are visible in this Indigenous subgroup, and the impacts on identity and identification, how the community perceives their own health risks, and how their specific cultural traditions prevent or respond to those risks can be examined. Emerging evidence about the protective role of cultural traditions, including Indigenous dance in mitigating the impacts of historical trauma on health outcomes in Indigenous communities provides an opportunity to explore this phenomenon (e.g., Fernandez, 2019; Gallo et al., 2009).

Specifically, researchers on this project worked with a Community Advisory Board (CAB) to develop and conduct the first alcohol and other drug use (AOD) and HIV risk needs assessment of MAI adults who currently or previously participated or were connected to Danza Mexica (DM), and live in two urban areas in distinct regions of the U.S. The needs assessment included questions regarding perceptions of AOD and HIV risk factors related to unique race/ethnicity, culture, and migration experiences as well as protective factors related to traditional cultural practices and community/social cohesion in the two urban MAI communities. This paper presents preliminary analyses from the AOD and HIV-specific questions. Overall, 80% (n = 16) of the participants identified AOD as a significant risk factor, and 60% (n = 12) perceived HIV to be a health concern in the broad MAI community. Using an Indigenous feminist framework, this research presents these risks understanding the need to develop meaningful interventions while also recognizing them as contextualized responses to the violence of historical and ongoing colonial heteropatriarchy (Beltrán, Alvarez, & Puga, 2020; Walters, Beltrán, Evans-Campbell, & Simoni, 2011; Walters & Simoni, 2002) as well as evidence of colonial survival. Importantly, the majority of the participants described specific teachings and traditional cultural practices from DM related to AOD and HIV prevention and response, emphasizing personal and cultural identity, community support, and healing, evidence of the strengths and decolonial strategies for health and well-being embedded in the DM community.

Who are Mexican American Indians?

According to the U.S. Census Bureau, Office of Management and Budget, American Indians and Alaska Native (AIAN) is defined as "a person having origins in any of the original peoples of North and South America (including Central America) and who maintains tribal affiliation or community attachment" (U.S. Census Bureau, 2020). MAI is a broad "tribal grouping" category that encompasses individuals living in the U.S. but with tribal affiliation or

attachment to Indigenous groups of Mexico. As with most racial/ethnic categories, identities are complex and intersectional. AIAN people may or may not
self-identify as Mexican/MAI, may self-identify as one or more racial/ethnic or
tribal categories, may have been born in the U.S., Mexico, or elsewhere and
may or may not be U.S. citizens, residents, or undocumented (Grieco et al.,
2012). People who self-identify within the MAI category may be descendants
or current members of Indigenous groups with protected status as defined by
constitutions within each Mexican state (Flannigan, 2016). Such groups may
include Maya, Zapotec, Otomi (Fox & Rivera-Salgado, 2004), Mixtec,
P'urhépecha, and Nahua (Ortiz, 2014). They may also descend from
Indigenous groups who are understood as ancestral predecessors of current
Indigenous groups such as Olmeca, Chichimeca, and Toltec (Colín, 2014).
Furthermore, they may be descendants or enrolled citizens of nations like the
Tohono O'odham, Yaqui, Kickapoo, and Kumeyaay – whose lands are divided
by the U.S./Mexico border (Starks et al., 2011).

These complex and intersectional identities are linked to diverse migration
histories, which include processes of ethnicization and identity formation that
may be influenced by community involvement and political actions. Historical
and contemporary oppression rooted in Spanish colonization within Mexican
society as well as contemporary oppression rooted in xenophobia in the
U.S. are common threads that link many individuals within this group
(Fernandez, 2019; Ortiz, 2014). These diverse and yet convergent histories
form the basis for the contemporary health status of MAI. Given both
a significant dearth of overall MAI health literature, yet similar historical and
contemporary colonial-based traumas, AOD, and HIV health literature drawn
from Latinx and AIAN populations can provide insight into health disparities,
risk, and protective factors among MAI (Zúñiga et al., 2014).

Historical trauma, AOD, and HIV

Over the last several decades, scholars have linked historical trauma to health
risk behaviors in AIAN communities (Duran & Walters, 2004; Evans-
Campbell, 2008; Evans-Campbell & Walters, 2006) and Mexican and
Mexican American communities (Estrada, 2009). Historical trauma is
defined as a collective and cumulative trauma experienced and transmitted
across generations resulting from devastating events targeting a community
(e.g., for AIAN, boarding schools, forced relocation, massacres; Brave Heart
et al., 2011; Brave Heart & DeBruyn, 1998; Evans-Campbell, 2008; Evans-
Campbell & Walters, 2006). In Mexican origin communities, historically
traumatic events subsequent to massacres and foreign disease that led to
significant population reduction in the entire Indigenous population of the
Americas (Dunbar-Ortiz, 2014) included the creation of a Spanish settler-
colonial state through the establishment of large ranches or plantations

sustained by forced Indigenous labor (Barajas, 2014; Estrada, 2009). Under the Treaty of Guadalupe Hidalgo in 1848, a large portion of what is now known as the southwestern U.S. was annexed to the U.S., further compounding oppression of Indigenous peoples living in this region (Barajas, 2014; Dunbar-Ortiz, 2014; Schulze, 2018). The Spanish developed a racialized caste system, increasing division and magnifying oppression of those who identified with and/or were phenotypically Indigenous (Dunbar-Ortiz, 2007; Estrada, 2009), in attempt to further unify and solidify Spanish political power driven by racialized nationalism (Estrada, 2009; J. Luna, 2013; J. M. Luna, 2011). The legacy of such colonial oppression continues through economic policies that are driving forces behind displacement and northern migration such as the North American Free Trade Agreement (NAFTA) (Castillo-Muñoz, 2013), the racism (Barajas, 2014) and xenophobia they face in the U.S. (Ortiz, 2014), as well as gender-based violence in both Mexico and the U.S. (Mirandé, 2016).

The effects of such exposure to historically traumatic events and intergenerational trauma are felt personally and collectively, and can result in high rates of mental health problems, substance abuse, and other health and social cohesion issues (Brave Heart et al., 2011; Evans-Campbell, 2008). The epidemiological literature on substance abuse and HIV among Latinos and AIAN raise particular concern about potential risk among MAI. Starting in early adolescence, Latinos and AIAN have the highest alcohol and illicit drug use in the country. AIAN communities tend to drink earlier, more heavily and frequently, and with more catastrophic outcomes than other groups (Walters et al., 2002). Additionally, Hispanic high school students reported the highest lifetime prevalence of ever having had an alcoholic drink, current alcohol use, and having had their first drink before the age of 13 when compared to White and Black peers (Center for Disease Control and Prevention [CDC], 2018).

Studies document high co-morbidity of AOD and HIV (Belani et al., 2012). Investigating HIV risk behaviors, Bertolli et al. (2004) found that the number of AIAN diagnosed with HIV who met the criteria for alcohol dependence was nearly twice the rate of non-AIAN counterparts. HIV rates in Hispanic/Latino and AIAN communities are also troubling. From 2010 to 2016, HIV diagnoses increased 46% in AIAN communities overall and 81% in gay and bisexual AIAN men (CDC, 2019b). In a 2019 Census Bureau estimate, Latinos represented 18.3% of the total U.S. population, yet accounted for 25% of new HIV infections in 2017 and rates of infection in Latinos were more than three times that of whites (CDC, 2019a, 2019c; U.S. Census Bureau, 2020).

There are a number of prevention challenges contributing to HIV shared by AIAN and Hispanic/Latino communities including cultural and socioeconomic factors, access to care, and HIV stigma (CDC, 2013; 2019b; 2019d), 2018a,). For Hispanic/Latino populations there are also factors related to language barriers, immigration status, and gender roles (CDC, 2013; 2019d).

For example, "*machismo*," the display of masculine characteristics, virility, and strength in men and, "*marianismo*," which conversely, requires sexual purity in women, as well as stigma associated with homosexuality are often described as challenges to HIV prevention among Latino/a communities (CDC, 2013; 2019d). Indigenous feminism understands these terms as social constructions which can place the blame and burden of responsibility for social and structural harm on individuals, communities, and cultural groups. Many Latin American scholars have described the term *machismo* as stereotyping and reductionist, racist in connotation, and overlooking the multiplicity and dynamic nature of masculinities (Goicolea et al., 2014). Such limited descriptions of gender roles can create cultural pathologies (Arvin et al., 2013; Mirandé, 2016; Torres et al., 2002) while also obscuring the impact of historical and ongoing colonialization and socio structural harm (Cripe, et al., 2015) on gender, sexuality and associated risk behaviors in Indigenous and Latinx communities.

Along with the existence of high rates of AOD, HIV, and other health risks and prevention challenges related to historical trauma, research has identified numerous protective mechanisms that may buffer the impact of trauma on AOD and HIV risk. Cultural resilience factors, which have shown promise in buffering the effects of traumatic stressors on health outcomes in AIAN communities, include enculturation (Novins et al., 2012; Walters et al., 2002), spirituality, and traditional health practices (Novins et al., 2012; Walters et al., 2002), and feelings of connection to family, community, and the environment (Evans-Campbell, 2008; Mohatt et al., 2011). Participation in Indigenous dance can form a "socially determined sense of place" (Ullrich, 2019, p. 4), which can be framed as a Native Hub (Ramirez, 2007), a transportable, potentially protective place wherein its practitioners can practice spiritual and cultural traditions that can strengthen and reinforce feelings of connection to family, community, and environment (Fernandez, 2019; Ramirez, 2007). Thus, participation in cultural dance can provide a sense of place wherein community can connect, practice traditions, and transmit knowledge based on Indigenous teachings about identity and health (Fernandez, 2019). For participants in this sample, Danza Mexica is a Native Hub wherein participants proactively decolonize and indigenize traditional understandings of substance use, health, and gender and sexuality.

What is Danza Mexica?[2]

Danza Mexica refers to dance traditions commonly rooted in pre-Cuauhtemoc ceremonies of Indigenous Nahuatl-speaking groups from Central Mexico. Participants in DM may trace biological and/or cultural roots to Mexica (Aztecs), who are considered to be Nahuatl-speaking ancestors of Indigenous groups of Mexico today (Colín, 2014). Originally migrating during the twelfth century from the Utah area of the U.S. Southwest to the current day Mexico City area, the Aztecs were known as one of several large, highly advanced, expansive civilizations that traded extensively with other civilizations and absorbed other local Indigenous nations (Dunbar-Ortiz, 2014). However, the Spanish colonial invasion brought genocide and multiple attacks on intellectual, cultural, spiritual, economic, and social systems not only of the Aztecs, but also of Indigenous nations throughout what is now known as Mexico (Colín, 2014; Fernandez, 2019; Luna, 2013; Sten, 1990).

Despite the physical and psychological attacks on their existence, practitioners of *danza* and other Indigenous traditions resisted and were able to maintain some of their practices underground, as well as through religious syncretism of *danza* with Catholic traditions as a testament to their resilience (Colín, 2014; J. Luna, 2013). There is a long and complex genealogy of Aztec Dance forms which have survived multiple colonizations (e.g., Spanish invasion, Mexican Nation-state sanctions and control) and migrations. As such, there are a variety of Aztec Dance forms practiced throughout Mexico, the U.S., and beyond that are nuanced and dynamic. For example, Conchero is a centuries old tradition that blends Catholic rites with Indigenous ceremonies. Mexicayotl is a more recent tradition focusing on a return to Native Indigenous practices in tandem with a decolonial approach to cultural diffusion and education. Tradición is a blend of Conchero and Mexicayotl values and practices (Colín, 2014). According to E. Lopez, "DM does not have one voice, one view or one belief... we are all flames of the same fire... unique, distinct, unified but not uniform (personal communication, May 19, 2020). Though there are many variations of traditions that continue to evolve and grow in nuanced ways, individuals in this study sample primarily participate in danza traditions most closely aligned with the Mexicayotl form to varying degrees. While it is important to note there are multiple other traditional ceremonial health-promoting practices that occur alongside DM (e.g., velacion/all-night vigil, temazcal/sweat lodge, tipi), the analysis presented here centers on participants' perceptions of DM specifically in relation to AOD and HIV prevention as they may be embedded in DM's holistic approach to health and healing.

Methods

Using a convenience sample approach and snowball strategy, we recruited 21 participants who identified as both Mexican (or Latino/Latina/Latinx of Mexican origin) and Indigenous adults (18 and over). They included men, women, and gender non-conforming (e.g., transgender, intersex, Two-Spirit, or tribally specific gender identity) individuals who participated (currently or previously) in DM. One participant who did not trace their Indigenous ancestry to Mexico was excluded from this analysis.

This needs assessment focused on obtaining participant perceptions of existing AOD, HIV, and other health needs in the MAI community broadly as well as cultural strengths in the MAI/DM community. We did not ask participants to describe their own AOD use or HIV status. We used digital-audio recording to capture in-depth interviews, which were conducted in both English and Spanish, depending on participant preference and lasted between 1 and 4 hours. Interviews were transcribed and translated by both professional transcriptionists and research staff, and then cleaned and de-identified. All transcripts were analyzed with Atlas.ti.

For thematic analysis, we created an initial codebook using the in-depth interview questionnaire to develop relevant thematic categories. After we had compiled and uploaded the data to our analytic software, we disassembled the data in the initial coding process. Initial coding reduced the data into distinct components for close examination, and then allowed for comparing and contrasting them with one another (Saldaña, 2009). After initial coding was complete, an in-depth analysis revealed sub-themes with more intricate meanings that shed light on the complexities of participant perceptions of AOD, HIV, and cultural strengths.

Results

The sample consists of 20 total participants including ten women, seven men, two trans women, and one who marked "other." Ages ranged from 18 to 55. Formal education level of participants ranged from none to a doctorate degree, with nine having earned a bachelor's degree or higher. To protect confidentiality, pseudonyms are used, and participants are broken into age cohorts (younger adult, adult, older adult). Gender is described as female/feminine and male/masculine to indicate that some participants were male- or female-identified, and others were transmasculine or transfeminine identified without singling out specific individuals. In this analysis, as participants use terms such as "machismo" or describe incidents of homophobia, these are understood as responses to the violence of colonial heteropatriarchy rather than characteristics attributable to individuals or cultural groups. Several participants describe them as "symptoms" of colonial trauma.

Race/ethnicity and Indigenous identity

It is important to note that self-identification categories are complex and often constructed by government bodies. Girón (2017) describes the challenges of getting an accurate population count within the category of Latin American Indian due to perceptions of the definition of American Indian as limited to tribes within the U.S. When asked about race/ethnic identity on the demographic questionnaire, 13 participants indicated they identified as Mexican/Latino, 5 did not respond, and 2 denied identifying this way. Almost every participant indicated a unique Indigenous or tribal heritage, with Mexica being the sole response for only two participants. Other responses included a combination of Mexica and P'urhépecha, Yaqui, Aztec, and Huichol. Mixteco, Ñuu Savi, Raramuri, Tarahumara, Cora, Otomi, Apache, and Chichimeca were also represented.

Alcohol and other drugs

Participants were asked to reflect on their perceptions of health needs and struggles within the MAI community broadly. Specifically, they were asked to reflect on whether alcohol and other drugs were concerns in the greater community, and what specific challenges they knew of in relation to those risks. Of the 20 participants interviewed, 80% (n = 16) believed that alcohol and other drugs were a concern in the MAI community. Among these discussions, two preliminary salient themes emerged: the socialization of AOD use, and AOD use as coping strategy, with a particular emphasis on alcohol use.

Socialization of substance use: a historical trauma response

While connection to culture is linked to reduced alcohol use for Indigenous Mexicans (Ozer & Fernald, 2008; Zúñiga et al., 2014), literature describing the patterns of alcohol abuse in developing countries such as Mexico (Medina-Mora, 2007) reveal the systemic influence of the colonial state on substance use in the MAI community. A number of participants described the normalization of substance use through the social experience in Mexico and in Mexican and Mexican American communities. Daisy, a female/fem., older adult, expressed concern that the socialization of substance use led to a lack of information about healthy and unhealthy patterns. For example, Daisy described her perceptions:

> The lack of education is what causes many of our people to not seek out help when they are in need. You don't become a drug addict or alcoholic overnight, it is a process. But, we don't recognize it because in our community alcohol is always present. You don't know that you are sick. So we don't ask for help until we are already in too deep.

In the Mexican health system, alcohol dependence is not considered a disease with corresponding treatment and public health campaigns to reduce problem drinking are scarce (Medina-Mora, 2007). For participants, struggles with alcohol use were linked to not only socialization experienced growing up in their communities, but also to gender roles. Angel, a younger male/masculine adult, described his perception of alcohol use as embedded in the broader Mexican community, particularly by males. He described the connection between the use of alcohol and *machismo*, and also began discussing the use of alcohol as a coping strategy or a "vice" that helps people get through difficult experiences. Angel said:

> Alcohol is a huge thing, because it's so embedded in our culture, in tequila and *machismo*; and I feel like a lot of dads – the majority – they drink a lot. They choose a vice … it could be eating junk food, it could be drinking alcohol, maybe cigarettes. But, for a lot of dads, they choose alcohol, because it's just always been there.

Mainstream alcohol research with Hispanic/Latino men attributes *machismo* to problem drinking behaviors (Fragoso & Kashubeck, 2000), but often without a clear description of the term (Perotte & Zamboanga, 2019). Historical trauma research describes alcohol use as one response to colonial violence (Braveheart, 2003; Brave Heart et al., 2011; Evans-Campbell, 2008). Likewise, gendered experiences associated with risky substance use behaviors can be understood as historical trauma responses to legacies of colonization, patriarchy, heteronormativity, and the systems that maintain them. Angel confirms this by further discussing how high rates of alcohol abuse and machismo are often described as part of Mexican culture but clarifies, "none of those things were part of our Native teachings. They exist because of the *removal* of our original teachings and [the Indigenous] value of community and collectivism."

Coping strategy and/or medicine for trauma

Similar to Angel's perceptions, and similar to other Indigenous peoples' use of alcohol to carry the pain of colonization (Brave Heart et al., 2011), several participants described AOD use as coping strategy to process emotional distress. Angel further explained, "A lot of people they're just not content, or they're not happy, with their lives. So, when they get home from work they want something's that's going take that away … And it's like … a medication. They self-medicate through alcohol." Another participant, Juana, also described AOD as a way to "medicate the hard things" and to survive daily hardships of life while Indigenous. She stated: "[I've seen] abuse of a lot of substances … It's very present because I think Indigenous people's lives are challenging" (Juana, adult, female/fem.). Similarly, Olivia, an adult female/fem. participant discussed the ways that she perceived poverty, lack of access to care, poor social support, and histories of genocide – factors associated with historical trauma – to impact AOD use. She explained:

> If you don't have healthy bonds, if you don't have the tools to build healthy relationships, if you don't have support in the community, your chances of

overcoming alcohol and drug addiction are super low. So, our communities have histories of genocide, we're in poverty, and we have no access to care. We don't have the resources, and we have higher rates of addiction. I think they're really connected. There's a lot of generational trauma and lack of resources that makes healthiness seem really impossible.

Teachings from Danza Mexica related to AOD

In addition to asking participants to reflect on challenges related to AOD in the MAI community, they were asked to reflect on resources and strategies that might exist within the community to help mitigate the risks. Specifically, the participants were asked to reflect on teachings from DM related to AOD use. Responses were clear that there are a number of teachings in DM related to clarity of mind, pride in identity, and healing through community and ceremonial practices. For example, *danzantes* (dancers) are encouraged to approach danza practice and ceremony with clear minds. Angel described the importance of "finding yourself" or finding "your way" in the practice of DM, which he described as challenging if one's clarity of mind is obscured by substances.

Typically, participation in DM *ensayos* (practices) or ceremonies prohibits active use of AOD; however, expectations for AOD abstinence or reduction vary between groups. Several participants described the AOD intervention possibilities embedded in DM. For example, Izel, a female/fem., adult, described the support that individuals receive from DM during struggles with AOD. She said:

> The medicine. The medicine from the dance, the circle, the prayers; all of the energy that we call the medicine, the act of being there in the circle. It is something that you cannot see, but it is there. Once you are in the circle and you feel this, you hear the drum and everything begins to move, it is like an energy medicine. And once you begin to dance, and you are singing, you are moving your body, it is like you are working towards this. ... If they come and ask to be better or to change their way of thinking or to find a better path, and if they are consistent, they will achieve this.

Some *danzantes* discussed their perceptions that AOD use in the community stemmed from internal issues including lack of self-worth, lack of connection to family, and lack of a strong personal identity. Adrian shared her perspective that DM is particularly powerful for addressing issues related to AOD in that it restores a sense of meaning and purpose in someone's life. Adrian, an older adult female/fem., shared:

> Drugs and alcohol ... I see those to be the problems that most affect the community. Those involved in the group that have connected and really know how to reap the benefits of Danza ... the benefits of belonging to a group, a *calpulli*,[3] a family, to transform their lives and leave behind alcohol and drugs, to have a purpose in life and identity, knowing where you come from, knowing that you have a past, and that you have a group that has your back and makes you feel that you have a future.

HIV risk and challenges in the community

Participants were asked to describe their perceptions of struggles or challenges with HIV in the MAI community. Overall, 60% (n = 12) believed that HIV was a concern in the MAI community. The overwhelming response from the participants was that the community does not discuss HIV, which some connected to stigma rooted in Catholicism, and others described as a lack of education and information about HIV.

"We don't talk about it"

Of the 12 who identified HIV as a concern in the community, 10 described variations of "we don't talk about it" as Mazatl, an adult male/masc. said. Most participants said this was true in the MAI community broadly but also within the DM community. Teresa, an older adult, female/fem. shared

> ... We don't talk about HIV. I can't think of a time ... that we talked about HIV. Except for once when some outside visitors were basically saying that Two Spirit people needed to be careful because of the risk for HIV, which didn't feel like a teaching, it felt like a judgement. ... This is where we have some decolonizing to do, because HIV has a lot to do with gender and sexuality, and also with substance use. We have a lot of room to grow in terms of teaching about it.

Several other participants discussed the perceived connection between *machismo* and the lack of conversations about HIV, healthy relationships, and sexual health among the DM community. Angel, young adult male/masc. described the different ways the information is communicated to and with the female/fem. members of the group compared to the (lack of) conversations among the male/masc. members of the group. He said:

> I know that [a female leader] has had talks with the girls in my group, not just those things, but also how to carry yourself as a woman and respect yourself, to set boundaries, to say 'no.' But on the male side ... it's never been talked about, and it may be a *machismo* type of thing. I think most of the time males in my community, not just the Danza circle, but I feel like there's this *machismo* arrogance that's like ... Like, 'we don't have to talk about it.'

Stigma rooted in Catholicism

Several participants described the lack of conversations and information in the MAI community about HIV and related health issues as rooted in the stigmas of homophobia and transphobia. Adrian, a female/fem., older adult described these roots in the community:

> HIV remains a condition with a lot of social stigma ... which is a result of the disinformation that spread when the epidemic first emerged. ... The way that it [HIV] is transmitted, if it is through sexual relations, and the fact that the group that it first developed in, the gay community, already had its own stigmas ... This disinformation remains in the minds of the people.

Other participants discussed the stigma as explicitly connected to the influence of Catholicism on beliefs and values. That is, even when Catholicism is not actively practiced, its influence as a primary component of the colonialization of Mexico and its people remains. Mazatl, adult male/masc., said, "We don't talk about it, because of the Catholic beliefs that we have in our own people. So, you have HIV, because you're in a sin. Therefore, god is punish[ing] you. So, we don't talk about it." Olivia, a female/fem. adult, agreed that the implicit connection between HIV and the Lesbian, Gay, Bisexual, Trans, Queer, Two-Spirit (LGBTQ2+) community, and the stigma of LGBTQ2+ identity within communities currently or historically influenced by Catholicism prevents conversations about HIV in the MAI community. She shared, "Maybe this topic gets tied into the stigma of sexuality … I think about it being connected to Mexican Indigenous culture and then Mexican culture being connected to Catholicism and the lessons [that you] don't talk about sexuality and sex."

Lack of education

Similar to the prevention challenges described earlier (CDC, 2013; CDC, 2019b; 2019d), misinformation, lack of access to resources, and an overall lack of education about HIV in the MAI and DM communities were perceived to be major blocks to preventing HIV risk among the community members. Some participants reflected on the need for educational materials about HIV and sexual health in Spanish and other languages. Others talked about the need to combat misinformation and stereotypes that have held on over time in the MAI community broadly as remnants of colonial hetero-patriarchy. Several participants expressed a need for the community to grow in order to be able to address HIV concerns. Juana, a female/fem. adult explained, "I think the community needs to grow. In order for that to happen, there needs to be education; proactive approaches to teaching people that HIV isn't this death sentence. There needs to be more knowledge and awareness." Mazatl, a male/masc., adult argued that there might be ways to think about traditional approaches to health and healing from HIV, but that the community needs to be ready to think about HIV without stereotypes and judgments. He said, "This is about helping each other. Maybe going back to our ways of curing people. And making them feel that just because they're [HIV] positive doesn't mean that they're evil. They're not contagious."

Teachings from Danza related to HIV

The participants were asked to discuss any teachings from DM related to HIV and sexual health. Several participants explained that while they could not name specific teachings from DM related to HIV, they felt that many of the underlying values and practices within DM such as community support, passing knowledge along to future generations, and the focus on healing traumas could support and facilitate conversations about HIV and sexual health. Gabriel, a male/masc. older adult asserted that helping one another and providing resources is one of the purposes of a DM community, and that it should be no different with regards to information about HIV. He said, "What we are doing in the group doesn't only have to do with issues relating to Danza, but this type of help as well and we try to have a bit of information to give them." Raúl, a male/masc. young adult reinforced this idea of community support as central to DM. He said, "We do that a lot when somebody is going through something like that, sit together and talk about it, 'how can we help you?' So you never feel like you're unwanted because we're a group, we're a family." Daisy, a female/fem. older adult, shared that she believes everything is connected to DM teachings about respect and knowledge and passing those values on to future generations. She said that this should include conversations about HIV, sexual health, and sexuality with children and young people. Rosamaria, a female/fem. adult agreed that including the younger generation in education about HIV was critical to preventing it and to reducing the stigma of the subject. Rosamaria said, "If we want to have a community or a society where it's not taboo to talk about HIV, and about protection and just Sex Ed in general, then who do we start with? We start with the kids."

Sergio, an adult male/masc. community member discussed the ways that DM teaches about healing, and the specific ways that these teachings can help community members with the health problems they are dealing with, including HIV. Sergio explained:

> My goal would be to heal them. And how do you heal people? You help them work through their traumas. When you become part of a [danza] community we're gonna help you get through whatever you're going through. Whether it's HIV ... alcoholism, whatever it is, we're gonna be there to support you and to help you feel good. Because once you start to feel good, you start to make better decisions ... you start to live better ... those things create this positive chain of events ... all this is a web.

Discussion

Findings from this needs assessment point to important AOD and HIV health concerns in the MAI community. Consistent with literature on HIV prevention challenges in populations who may fall within the MAI category, participant perceptions suggest high rates of alcohol and other drug abuse within the MAI community broadly, as well as silence and stigma around HIV and sexual health that is of concern. Simultaneously, the teachings embedded in DM's holistic approach to health and healing highlight strengths, unique cultural strategies, and decolonial practices that may facilitate protection from these risks. Emphasizing clarity of mind, strong personal and cultural identity, and community support to navigate and heal from trauma, it is clear that the teachings from DM contribute culture-centered approaches to health for the MAI community.

As the first of its kind, this needs assessment contributes uniquely to the literature about AOD and HIV within Indigenous communities. However, limitations of this study include the small sample size and the singular focus on the subgroup of DM within the MAI community, reducing generalizability to the MAI population as a whole, and to Indigenous communities of the U.S. The participants within the sample had higher levels of education than is common within this population, and suggests a potential skew in the data. It must also be considered whether members of DM are a meaningful subgroup within the MAI community, particularly due to the historically political nature of the DM community as well as the diversity between group beliefs and practices. Additional research within the DM, and more broadly within the MAI community should explore complexities of the MAI community, including generational differences, and the experiences of community members with intersectional identities.

Conclusion

There is a dearth of research focusing on the MAI community. As the population continues to grow and self-identify, further research is needed to examine the specific needs and strengths of the MAI community. To advance this agenda, this research identified the subgroup of MAI community members who participate in Danza Mexica as uniquely situated to describe the ways that cultural practices can be utilized to inform prevention and intervention efforts. It is clear that while there are AOD and HIV concerns within the MAI broadly, there are also culture-centered beliefs, values, and practices embedded in DM tradition preventive of AOD use which are endemic to the tradition. Additionally, there is room to grow in terms of using DM beliefs, values, and practices to leverage cultural knowledge and decolonize stigma around gender, sex, sexuality, and HIV. Specifically, participants in this sample described opportunities to incorporate HIV-specific and sexual health information to the culture of support that already exists within the DM traditions. These preliminary findings have the potential to contribute to the development of culturally relevant and decolonial prevention and treatment approaches that are sustainable for the MAI community to reduce AOD and HIV disparities and promote overall community health and wellness.

Notes

1. The term "Mexican American Indian" emerges from the race/ethnic categories defined by the U.S. government in official census reports and, as evidenced by data represented in this paper, is not a term that the community uses for self-identification. For purposes of clarity, we use the term in this paper to describe the population included in our sample.
2. Colín (2014) describes the many "regional, ontological and organizational" (p. 224) descriptions of this practice including "*Danza Conchera, Danza Mexica, Danza Azteca,*

Tradición, Danza Azteca-Chichimeca, Chitontequiza, Macehualiztli, Mitotilitzli, and beyond … (p. 224)." In contemporary vernacular and particularly in the U.S., *Azteca* and *Mexica* are used interchangeably (Colín, 2014). We use the term *Danza Mexica* because it is what the majority of our participants used to describe their traditions. We also use *danza* as shorthand.

3. Calpulli is a Nahuátl word stemming from the words *calli* (house) and *pulli* (reunion). In danza, the term can be understood as a "union of houses" or an alliance between families and most commonly describes the danza group as it works together (Colín, 2014).

Acknowledgments

Research reported in this publication was supported by the National Institute of Mental Health of the National Institutes of Health under Award Number R25MH084565. The content is solely the responsibility of the authors and does not necessarily represent the official views of the National Institutes of Health. The authors extend our deep gratitude to community leaders and community members for guiding us through this research, welcoming us into their homes and sacred spaces, and for sharing their important stories. We raise our hands to you.

Disclosure statement

No potential conflict of interest was reported by the authors.

ORCID

Angela R. Fernandez ⓘ http://orcid.org/0000-0001-9066-7367

References

Arvin, M., Tuck, E., & Morrill, A. (2013). Decolonizing feminism: Challenging connections between settler colonialism and heteropatriarchy. *Feminist Formations, 25*(1), 8–34. https://doi.org/10.1353/ff.2013.0006

Barajas, M. (2014). Colonial dislocations and incorporation of Indigenous migrants from Mexico to the United States. *American Behavioral Scientist, 58*(1), 53–63. https://doi.org/10.1177/0002764213495031

Belani, H., Chorba, T., Fletcher, F., Hennessey, K., Kroeger, K., Lansky, A., … O'Connor, K. (2012). Integrated prevention services for HIV infection, viral hepatitis, sexually transmitted diseases, and tuberculosis for persons who use drugs illicitly: Summary guidance from CDC and the US Department of Health and Human Services. *Morbidity and Mortality Weekly Report: Recommendations and Reports, 61*(5), 1–43. https://www.cdc.gov/mmwr/preview/mmwrhtml/rr6105a1.htm

Beltrán, R, Alvarez, A, & Madrid-Puga, M. (2020). Morning Star, Sun, and Moon Share the Sky: (Re)membering Two Spirit Identity through Culture-Centered HIV Prevention Curriculum for Indigenous Youth. In Nickel, S., & Fehr, A. (Eds.). (2020). In Good Relation: History, Gender, and Kinship in Indigenous Feminisms. Univ. of Manitoba Press.

Bertolli, J., McNaghten, A. D., Campsmith, M., Lee, L. M., Leman, R., Bryan, R. T., & Buehler, J. W. (2004). Surveillance systems monitoring HIV/AIDS and HIV risk behaviors among American Indians and Alaska Natives. *AIDS Education and Prevention*, *16*(3), 218–237. https://doi.org/10.1521/aeap.16.3.218.35442

Brave Heart, M. Y., Chase, J., Elkins, J., & Altschul, D. B. (2011). Historical trauma among Indigenous peoples of the Americas: Concepts, research, and clinical considerations. *Journal of Psychoactive Drugs*, *43*(4), 282–290. https://doi.org/10.1080/02791072.2011.628913

Brave Heart, M. Y., & DeBruyn, L. M. (1998). The American Indian holocaust: Healing historical unresolved grief. *American Indian and Alaska Native Mental Health Research*, *8* (2), 56–78. https://doi.org/10.5820/aian.0802.1998.60

Brave Heart, M. Y. H. (2003). The historical trauma response among natives and its relationship with substance abuse: a lakota illustration. *Journal of Psychoactive Drugs*, *35*(1), 7-13. https://doi.org/10.1080/02791072.2003.10399988

Castillo-Muñoz, V. (2013). Historical roots of rural migration: Land reform, corn credit, and the displacement of rural farmers in Nayarit Mexico, 1900–1952. *Mexican Studies/Estudios Mexicanos*, *29*(1), 36–60. https://doi.org/10.1525/msem.2013.29.1.36

Center for Disease Control and Prevention. (2018). *Youth risk behaviour surveillance — United States, 2017.* Center for Surveillance, Epidemiology, and Laboratory Services, Centers for Disease Control and Prevention. https://www.cdc.gov/healthyyouth/data/yrbs/pdf/2017/ss6708.pdf

Centers for Disease Control. (2013, November). *HIV among Hispanics/Latinos in the United States and dependent areas.* http://www.hivlawandpolicy.org/sites/default/files/HIV%20Among%20Hispanics.pdf

Centers for Disease Control and Prevention. (2018a). *HIV Surveillance Report, 2017* (Vol. 29). http://www.cdc.gov/hiv/library/reports/hiv-surveillance.html

Centers for Disease Control and Prevention. (2019a). Diagnoses of HIV Infection in the United States and Dependent Areas, 2018 (Preliminary). https://www.cdc.gov/hiv/pdf/library/reports/surveillance/cdc-hiv-surveillance-report-2018-preliminary-vol-30.pdf

Centers for Disease Control and Prevention. (2019b). HIV and American Indians and Alaska natives. Retrieved from: https://www.cdc.gov/hiv/pdf/group/racialethnic/aian/cdc-hiv-aian-fact-sheet.pdf

Centers for Disease Control and Prevention. (2019c). HIV in the United States and Dependent Areas [Fact Sheet]. https://www.cdc.gov/hiv/statistics/overview/ataglance.html

Centers for Disease Control and Prevention. (2019d). HIV and Hispanics/Latinos [Fact Sheet]. Retrieved from: https://www.cdc.gov/hiv/pdf/group/racialethnic/hispaniclatinos/cdc-hiv-latinos.pdf

Colín, E. T. (2014). *Indigenous education through dance and ceremony: A Mexica palimpsest.* Palgrave Macmillan.

Cripe, S. M., Espinoza, D., Rondon, M. B., Jimenez, M. L., Sanchez, E., Ojeda, N., ... & Williams, M. A. (2015). Preferences for intervention among Peruvian women in intimate partner violence relationships. Hispanic health care international: the official journal of the National Association of Hispanic Nurses, 13(1), 27. 10.1891/1540-4153.13.1.27

Dunbar-Ortiz, R. (2007). *Roots of resistance: A history of land tenure in New Mexico.* University of Oklahoma Press.

Dunbar-Ortiz, R. (2014). *An Indigenous people's history of the United States.* Beacon Press.

Duran, B., & Walters, K. L. (2004). HIV/AIDS prevention in "Indian Country": Current practice, indigenist etiology models, and postcolonial approaches to change. *AIDS Education & Prevention*, *16*(3), 187–201. https://doi.org/10.1521/aeap.16.3.187.35441

Estrada, A. (2009). Mexican-Americans and historical trauma theory: A theoretical perspective. *Journal of Ethnicity in Substance Abuse*, *8*(3), 330–340. https://doi.org/10.1080/15332640903110500

Evans-Campbell, T., & Walters, K. L. (2006). Indigenist practice competencies in child welfare practice: A decolonization framework to address family violence and substance abuse among First Nations peoples. InFong, R., McRoy, R., & Hendricks, C. (Eds.), Intersecting child welfare, substance abuse, and family violence: Culturally competent approaches (266-290). Council on Social Work Education.

Evans-Campbell, T. (2008). Historical trauma in American Indian/Native Alaska communities: A multilevel framework for exploring impacts on individuals, families, and communities. *Journal of Interpersonal Violence, 23*(3), 316–338. https://doi.org/10.1177/0886260507312290

Fernandez, A. R. (2019). *"Wherever I go, I have it inside of me": Indigenous cultural dance as a transformative place of health and prevention for members of an urban Danza Mexica community* [Doctoral dissertation]. Retrieved from Name of database. (Accession or Order Number)

Flannigan, S.I. (2016). Clarifying limbo: Disentangling Indigenous autonomy from the Mexican constitutional order. Perspectives on Federalism, 8(1),36–52. https://doi.org/10.1515/pof-2016-0003

Fox, J., & Rivera-Salgado, G. (2004). *Indigenous Mexican migrants in the United States.* University of California, San Diego, Center for U.S.-Mexican Studies, Center for Comparative Immigration Studies.

Fragoso, J. M., & Kashubeck, S. (2000). Machismo, gender role conflict, and mental health in Mexican American men. *Psychology of Men & Masculinity, 1*(2), 87–97. https://doi.org/10.1037/1524-9220.1.2.87

Gallo, L. C., Penedo, F. J., Espinosa de Los Monteros, K., & Arguelles, W. (2009). Resiliency in the face of disadvantage: Do Hispanic cultural characteristics protect health outcomes? *Journal of Personality, 77*(6), 1707–1746. https://doi.org/10.1111/j.1467-6494.2009.00598.x

Goicolea, I., Coe, A.-B., & Ohman, A. (2014). Easy to oppose, difficult to propose: Young activist men's framing of alternative masculinities under the hegemony of machismo in Ecuador. *YOUNG, 22*(4), 399–419. https://doi.org/10.1177/1103308814548109

Grieco, E. M., Acosta, Y. D., de la Cruz, G. P., Gambino, C., Gryn, T., Larsen, L. J., ... Walters, N. P. (2012). *The foreign-born population in the United States: 2010.* https://www.census.gov/prod/2012pubs/acs-19.pdf

Luna, J. (2013). La tradicion conchera: Historical process of Danza and Catholicism. *Dialogo, 16*(1), 47–64. https://doi.org/10.1353/dlg.2013.0000

Luna, J. M. (2011). *Danza Mexica: Indigenous identity, spirituality, activism, and performance* [Doctoral dissertation]. University of California. http://scholarworks.sjsu.edu/mas_pub/?utm_source=scholarworks.sjsu.edu%2Fmas_pub%2F1&utm_medium=PDF&utm_campaign=PDFCoverPages

Medina-Mora, M. E. (2007). Mexicans and alcohol: Patterns, problems and policies. *Addiction, 102*(7), 1041–1045. https://doi.org/10.1111/j.1360-0443.2007.01857.x

Mirandé, M. (2016). Hombres mujeres. *Men and Masculinities, 19*(4), 384–409. https://doi.org/10.1177/1097184X15602746

Mohatt, N. V., Fok, C. C. T., Burket, R., Henry, D., & Allen, J. (2011). Assessment of awareness of connectedness as a culturally-based protective factor for Alaska native youth. *Cultural Diversity and Ethnic Minority Psychology, 17*(4), 444. https://doi.org/10.1037/a0025456

Norris, T., Vines, P. L., & Hoeffel, E. M. (2012). The American Indian and Alaska native population: 2010. *2010 Census Briefs. U.S. Census Bureau.* Retrieved November 2012, from http://www.census.gov/prod/cen2010/briefs/c2010br-10.pdf

Novins, D. K., Boyd, M. L., Brotherton, D. T., Fickenscher, A., Moore, L., & Spicer, P. (2012). Walking on: Celebrating the journeys of Native American adolescents with substance use problems on the winding road to healing. *Journal of Psychoactive Drugs, 44*(2), 153–159. https://doi.org/10.1080/02791072.2012.684628

Ortiz, L. V. (2014). Transnational ethnic processes: Indigenous Mexican migrations to the United States. *Latin American Perspectives, 41*(3), 54–74. https://doi.org/10.1177/0094582X14532073

Ozer, E. J., & Fernald, L. C. H. (2008). Alcohol and tobacco use among rural Mexican adolescents: Individual, familial, and community level factors. *Journal of Adolescent Health, 43*(5), 498–505. https://doi.org/10.1016/j.jadohealth.2008.04.014

Perrotte, J. K, & Zamboanga, B. L. (2019). Traditional gender roles and alcohol use among latinas/os: a review of the literature. *Journal of Ethnicity in Substance Abuse, 1-18.* https://doi.org/10.1080/15332640.2019.1579142

Ramirez, R. K. (2007). *Native hubs: Culture, community, and belonging in Silicon Valley and beyond.* Duke University Press.

Saldaña, J. (2009). *Qualitative coding manual for qualitative researchers.* Thousand Oaks, CA: Sage.

Sandoval Girón, A. B. (2017). Central and South American Indigenous, American Indian or Hispanic/Latino Respondents? Navigating racial identity categories in U.S. Census Forms. Center for Survey Measurement, U.S. Census Bureau. Retrieved from: https://www.census.gov/content/dam/Census/newsroom/press-kits/2017/aapor/2017-aapor-sandoval.pdf

Schulze, J. M. (2018). *Are we not foreigners here? Indigenous nationalism in the U.S.-Mexico borderlands.* University of North Carolina Press.

Starks, R. R., McCormack, J., & Cornell, S. (2011). *Native nations and U.S. Borders.* The University of Arizona, Udall Center for Studies in Public Policy.

Sten, M. (1990). *Ponte a bailar, tu que reinas: antropologia de danza prehispanica.* Mexico City, Mexico: Editorial Joaquin Mortiz.

Torres, J., Solberg, V., & Carlstrom, A. (2002). The myth of sameness among Latino men and their machismo. *American Journal of Orthopsychiatry, 72*(2), 163–181. https://doi.org/10.1037/0002-9432.72.2.163

Ullrich, J. S. (2019). For the love of our children: An indigenous connectedness framework. *AlterNative: An International Journal of Indigenous Peoples, 15*(2), 121-130. https://doi.org/10.1177/1177180119828114

U.S. Census Bureau (2020, April). Race. Retrieved from https://www.census.gov/topics/population/race/about.html

United States Census Bureau. (2020). QuickFacts United States [Fact Sheet]. https://www.census.gov/quickfacts/fact/table/US/RHI725218

Walters, K. L., Simoni, J. M., & Evans-Campbell, T. (2002). Substance abuse among American Indians and Alaska natives: Incorporating culture in an "indigenist" stress-coping model. *Public Health Reports, 117*(Suppl. 1), 5104–5117. PMID: PMC1913706

Walters, K. L., & Simoni, J. M. (2002). Reconceptualizing Native women's health: An "indigenist" stress-coping model. American Journal of Public Health, 92(4),520–524. https://ajph.aphapublications.org/doi/abs/10.2105/AJPH.92.4.520

Walters, K.L, Beltrán, R. E, Evans-Campbell, T, & Simoni, J.M. (2011). Keeping our hearts from touching the ground: hiv/aids in american indian and alaska native women. *Women's Health Issues, 21-25,* S261-S265. doi: 10.1016/j.whi.2011.08

Zúñiga, M. L., Fischer, P. L., Cornelius, D., Cornelius, W., Goldenberg, S., & Keyes, D. (2014). A transnational approach to understanding indicators of mental health, alcohol use and reproductive health among indigenous Mexican migrants. *Journal of Immigrant and Minority Health, 16*(3), 329–339. https://doi.org/10.1007/s10903-013-9949-

Migration and resilience in Native Hawaiian elders

Kathryn L. Braun ⓘ, Colette V. Browne, Shelley Muneoka, Tyran Terada,
Rachel Burrage ⓘ, Yan Yan Wu ⓘ, and Noreen Mokuau

ABSTRACT
Using focused ethnography, Native Hawaiian elders living
away from Hawai'i for 30+ years were recruited through
Hawaiian organizations and word-of-mouth and interviewed
by teleconferencing on reasons for migrating, experiences on
the Continent, and resilience. The 18 participants in 13 states
left for college, work, and family. Many experienced racism, but
all created community and cultivated aloha in their new
homes. Most planned to stay on the Continent, although two-
thirds wanted remains/cremains returned to Hawai'i. Family,
culture, and financial well-being were sources of resilience.
Social workers should advocate for improved socioeconomic
and deracialized conditions for all people, and base interventions on cultural strengths.

Much of what we know about Native Hawaiians has been generated from
data collected in the Hawaiian Archipelago, the homeland of Native
Hawaiians. However, 45% of Native Hawaiians now live outside of the
state of Hawai'i (U.S. Census, 2012). This focused ethnography aimed to
hear from Native Hawaiians aged 60 or older who have lived 30 or more
years on the Continental US, with a particular interest in their reasons for
leaving, their experiences with aging and caregiving away from the islands,
and resilience factors.

The 2010 U.S. Census reported that 527,077 of the nation's citizens claim
Native Hawaiian ancestry, alone or in combination with other ethnicities
(U.S. Census, 2012). Native Hawaiians live in all 50 U.S. states, with the
largest concentrations in Hawai'i (55%), California, Washington, Nevada,
Texas, Oregon, Arizona, Florida, and Utah. Data from Hawai'i suggest that

Native Hawaiians have a shorter life expectancy and poorer health profiles compared to the state's largest racial/ethnic groups, including Japanese, Chinese, Filipino, and White (Wu et al., 2017). However, little is known about the Native Hawaiians who leave the state, their reasons for leaving, their experiences on the Continent, or how their departure influences aging and caregiving options and preferences.

Thinking about why Native Hawaiians migrate to other states is informed by theories of migration, which are commonly based in the concept of push and pull factors (Piché, 2013). Push factors include negative or unfavorable conditions in one's homeland, and pull factors are positive or favorable conditions in another community that motivate one to migrate. Migration also is influenced by economic disparities between communities, personal skills, gender, age, communication technology (which increases one's knowledge of other places and links to people living there), and social connections (e.g., migration is easier if you are following family or friends who migrated earlier).

The Native Hawaiian migration experience also may be informed by minority stress theory, which postulates that minority groups experience chronic stress due to racism, and this stress generates psychological and physiological responses that accumulate over time to produce poor health outcomes (Brandolo et al., 2009; Meyer, 2003; Pearlin et al., 2005; Sotero, 2006). Stressors that commonly effect indigenous peoples are grounded in their experience with colonization and include historical trauma, interpersonal bias, institutional racism, and financial insecurity (Braveheart & Debruyn, 1998; Stanley et al., 2017).

The Native Hawaiian population of Hawai'i declined by more than 80% in the first 100 years following European contact in 1778 due to exposure to introduced germs, guns, and alcohol (Merry, 2000). Although U.S. missionaries and businessmen were not the first Westerners in Hawai'i, within 50 years of their arrival they had worked together to gain control of the economy. Subsistence fishing and farming were largely replaced by extractive capitalist ventures of sugar and pineapple plantations. More than 300,000 laborers were imported from China, Portugal, Japan, Korea, the Philippines, and elsewhere to work the fields as Hawaiians died off, while the products of their labor were exported abroad. With the backing of the U.S. military, the Hawaiian monarchy of Queen Lili'uokalani was overthrown in 1893 and, despite opposition from the majority of the Hawaiian people, the islands were illegally annexed by the U.S. in 1898. Forced assimilation to American laws, language, culture, and religion followed, including criminal consequences for those who resisted (Goodyear-Ka'opua et al., 2014; Merry, 2000). Overt discrimination and micro-aggressions continue today (Sue et al., 2007). In research in Hawai'i, Kaholokula (2014) found that 48% of Native Hawaiians felt discriminated against "often" to "most of the time," while 52% experienced discrimination "sometimes" over a 12-month period.

Minority populations also have resilience-based factors, including cultural norms, values, traditions, and collective community, to help cope with stressors and their consequences. (Hausmann etal., 2010; Kirmayer etal., 2000). Resilience is recognized as important to the mental health of migrants, especially those that cross international borders (Siriwardhana etal., 2014). Resiliency factors for Native Hawaiians include astrong emphasis on family and cultural values and practices (Browne etal., 2009). Delegitimized for more than acentury by those who colonized Hawai'i, these cultural values have reemerged as asource of resilience and have been found to improve health and well-being when built into program interventions (Ka'opua etal., 2011; Mokuau etal., 2012).

This study was sponsored by Hā Kūpuna National Resource Center for Native Hawaiian Elders at the Myron B. Thompson School of Social Work, University of Hawai'i at Mānoa. Hā Kūpuna means the sharing of hā, (the breath of life, from kūpuna (elders) to younger generations. Established in 2006 with funding from the Administration on Community Living, U.S. Department of Health and Human Services, Hā Kūpuna is one of three congressionally mandated resource centers focusing on the health and long-term care needs and preferences of native elders (Browne et al., 2015). The mission of Hā Kūpuna is to generate knowledge about Native Hawaiian elders and enhance culturally competent long-term and supportive services. Our work is guided by an advisory council comprised of experts in gerontology and/or Hawaiian health; 80% of members are Native Hawaiian (Mokuau et al., 2008).

In terms of positionality, the investigators have a long-standing commitment to research, community capacity building, and policy development to improve indigenous health in Hawai'i and elsewhere. Much of the research on indigenous peoples presents data on the disparities they experience. Although these disparities are real and stem from the direct and lasting effects of colonization, pointing out disparities is often perceived by indigenous communities as "more bad news." Hā Kūpuna has taken a balanced approach to research, and this project was among those that aimed to document cultural strengths and factors that promote native resilience and health (Braun et al., 2014; Browne et al., 2009). Also, as gerontologists, we were interested in implications of the Hawaiian diaspora on aging and eldercare, as migration often splits families and reduces home care options.

The purpose of this study was to learn more about Native Hawaiian elders who lived and aged away from the islands. An earlier review of U.S. Census data by Hā Kūpuna suggested that kūpuna on the Continent may have higher socioeconomic status than kūpuna in Hawai'i (Nakatsuka et al., 2013). An earlier qualitative study, conducted among Native Hawaiian elders living in Southern California, found that discrimination was a factor in their migration from Hawai'i, but was less of a problem in their new communities. Participants identified challenges associated with aging and caregiving, and reflected how Native Hawaiian cultural traditions and values continued to shape their caregiving and service preferences (Browne & Braun, 2017). In the current study, we endeavored to hear from Native Hawaiian elders from across the nation. We were particularly interested in the push and pull factors that triggered their migration, their positive and negatives experiences living elsewhere, their experiences with parental care, plans for their own aging, and resilience factors that sustained them in their new homes.

Method

Study design

We conducted a focused ethnography to answer our research questions. This method is based in ethnography, an approach initially developed by anthropologists to learn about the beliefs, norms, structures, and artifacts of a culture through firsthand experience (Creswell & Poth, 2018). A focused ethnography is guided by specific research questions and conducted within a specific group and context (Mayan, 2009). This method often is used to learn enough about a select group to inform the tailoring of an intervention to increase its attractiveness to and accessibility by the group (Wainberg et al., 2007). This study was approved by the Institutional Review Board of the University of Hawai'i.

Participants

Individuals eligible to participate were age 60 or older and of Native Hawaiian ancestry, and must have lived away from the islands for 30 or more years. We worked with our advisory council members and established Hawaiian groups to identify eligible candidates. Of primary assistance was the Association of Hawaiian Civic Clubs, a confederation of 58 Hawaiian Civic Clubs located throughout Hawai'i and in many other states across the nation. The Native Hawaiian Civic Club movement was started in 1918 by Prince Jonah Kūhiō Kalaniana'ole, a member of the royal family and a delegate from Hawai'i to the U.S. House of Representatives, to help elevate Native Hawaiians through education and civic engagement. Researchers discussed the project with Civic Club leaders on the Continent, who could decide to forward (or not) our recruitment flyer to their members. One study participant volunteered after seeing a notice on the Kamehameha Schools Alumni Association blog. Others were recruited through personal networks of advisory council members, the research team, and research participants. Efforts were made to obtain an equal number of male and female participants and to hear from participants across the Continent. After the first dozen interviews, interviewers were hearing many of the same themes, indicating that thematic saturation had been reached; however, we decided to interview all individuals who already had consented to participate.

Data collection procedures

A short questionnaire was used to obtain background information on participants, including gender, age, marital status, educational attainment, and self-rated health. As appropriate for focused ethnography, interviews were led by a specific set of questions (Mayan, 2009). The interview started with questions about the participant's Hawaiian family names and places in the islands. Then the interviewer asked questions in five areas: reasons for leaving Hawai'i, advantages and disadvantages of living away from Hawai'i, racism as a push or pull factor, aging and caregiving away from the islands, and resilience factors. The interview schedule was designed by Native Hawaiian and non-Hawaiian members of the research team and pretested with two Native Hawaiian kūpuna.

The first three authors conducted interviews between March 2018 and February 2019. One of the interviewers was Native Hawaiian. By profession, two were licensed social workers, and the third was a public health researcher focusing on indigenous and immigrant health. The three interviewers completed an interview together to assure consistency in explaining the study, asking questions, and demonstrating cultural humility. The next seven interviews were done in pairs, and finally the first and third authors each conducted five interviews alone.

Once possible participants were identified, they were contacted by phone or e-mail to fully explain the study and asked if they would like to participate. If agreeable, they were sent and asked to return the consent form and background datasheet electronically or by mail in a pre-addressed, stamped envelope. Once the signed consent form was returned, a mutually convenient time was arranged for the interview; 15 interviews were conducted using teleconferencing technology, and three were in-person. Consent forms and background datasheets were stored in the locked program office in a locked cabinet. Relevant electronic files were stored on a password encrypted computer. Participants were informed that pseudonyms would be used and demographic details reported in aggregate to obscure individual identities. With permission, conversations were recorded. Interviews typically lasted 60 to 90 minutes. Audio records were transcribed, and both oral and written accounts of the interview were returned to participants, who could correct them and then keep the final copies for their files. Participants also received a thank you note and a 5 USD gift certificate to a sundry store.

Data processing and analysis

Latent content analysis was used to analyze data (Mayan, 2009). Prior to data analysis, the first author read and reread transcripts from the 13 interviews she conducted or co-conducted and drafted a codebook, which included detailed codes under the five broader thematic areas of interest (reasons for leaving and staying away, advantages and disadvantages of living away from Hawai'i, racism as a push or pull factor, aging and caregiving, and resilience and advice). Five members of the research team then used the draft codebook to code one interview. Although interrater reliability was high (r = 0.80), the discussion led to the refinement of some of the codes to better capture the wide range of experiences of the participants. For example, the code for experienced racism was split into four codes – personally experienced racism in Hawai'i, witnessed racism in Hawai'i, personally experienced racism on the continent, and witnessed racism on the continent. This final codebook was used to code all the interviews. The first author coded all 18 interviews, and four other members of the team each coded four or five transcripts, so that each transcript was coded by at least two people. Coders also highlighted passages that were particularly illustrative of a theme. Codes were entered into a spreadsheet that linked a participant's mention of a construct to the relevant page number in the transcript. This allowed us to check consistency in coding, to count codes, to review transcript snippets related to a code to understand nuances in participant experience, and to identify illustrative quotes.

Participants were invited to review the draft manuscript as a form of member checking (Mayan, 2009). We asked them to check quotes extracted from their transcripts to assure that information was not taken out of context and privacy was respected, and we asked for their agreement with the findings. Twelve of 18 (67%) responded, approving the manuscripts conclusions and sending comments. A few comments corrected or contextualized quotes or nuanced findings, and these were incorporated in subsequent revisions.

Rigor

Engaging multiple team members in interviewing and coding helped enrich perspectives on the data and reduce systematic bias, strengthening dependability of the findings. As interviews were completed and the data were coded, the team reflected on the themes at monthly meetings, and reflections helped to increase the confirmability of the data. In the data analysis and reporting stages of the research, inconsistencies and consistencies between the data and findings were discussed. Other efforts to increase credibility of the findings included interviewing until saturations, member checking, and attention to context. Findings appear to have high transferability, as they aligned with what is known about other migrant and minority groups (Mayan, 2009). Finally, two coauthors assessed the manuscript against the 21-item checklist from the Standards for Reporting of Qualitative Research to assure that necessary detail was provided in the introduction, methods, results, and discussion of the paper (O'Brien et al., 2014).

Results

Participants

Sixteen of the 18 participants were interviewed in their homes on the U.S. Continent, and two more, who had spent 30+ years in Colorado and Louisiana, respectively, were interviewed in Hawai'i. Their ages ranged from the early 60s to the mid-80s, 17 had attended college, and none rated their health as poor (Table 1). All participants could trace their ancestry back three or more generations and related proud stories of their forbearers' roles in Hawaiian history. All had one or more non-Hawaiian ancestors, usually of Chinese, Japanese, Filipino, Portuguese, or Caucasian descent. Several traced their ancestry to a specific community or ahupua'a (a uniquely Hawaiian geographical and political delineation of land). For example, by way of introduction, a woman who had lived away for more than 50 years said, "My mountain is Hualalai. My ahupua'a is Kawanui. My water is Keauhou Bay ... I can go back five, six generations. That's who I am."

Thematic areas

As appropriate for focused ethnography, where participants are responding to a structured set of questions, findings are presented within the five question categories, including reasons for leaving and staying away, advantages and disadvantages of living away from Hawai'i, racism as a push or pull factor, aging and caregiving, and resilience and advice.

Reasons for leaving and staying abroad

When asked about reasons for leaving Hawai'i, 14 said they wanted to leave, either temporarily or permanently, to expand their horizons and/or pursue adventure. For example, one said, "I just wanted something more." Another said, "I always wanted to work in New York." A woman said, "I studied hard so I could get a scholarship to go to college on the mainland." Another said, "I heard of better wages there and said 'why not try?'" Among the other four participants, one was born on the Continent (his Caucasian grandfather had married in Hawai'i and taken his Hawaiian bride to the Continental U.S.), and three migrated as children with their parents who followed work

Table 1. Demographics of the sample (n = 18).

Characteristic	N (%)
Living (or lived) in	
Arizona	2
California	2
Colorado	1
Florida	1
Illinois	1
Louisiana	1
Missouri	1
Nevada	1
New York	1
Oregon	1
Texas	1
Washington, DC	1
Washington	4
Gender	
Male	9 (50)
Female	9 (50)
Age group	
60s	6 (33)
70s	9 (50)
80s	3 (17)
Education attainment	
High school	1 (6)
Some college	5 (28)
BA/BS degree	6 (33)
Graduate degree	6 (33)
Marital status	
Married or Partnered	10 (56)
Other	8 (44)
Living arrangements	
With others	14 (78)
Alone	4 (22)
Self-rated health	
Excellent or very good	5 (28)
Good	8 (44)
Poor	5 (28)

opportunities. For example, one's father worked for the U.S. Post Office and was transferred, and another's father was a saddle maker who moved to Los Angeles to make saddles and tack for cowboys featured in western television shows and movies.

Of those who migrated as adults, six left to attend college, six joined the military, and two left for other work. Of those leaving for work, one secured employment on oil rigs in Louisiana. The other was invited by friends to work in Las Vegas, then joined a touring theater company, and ended up with a successful career in New York City. The individuals who joined the military tended to train in California or the U.S. South, and they served in Vietnam, Germany, Hawai'i, Texas, Washington, and other U.S. states.

Ten returned to Hawai'i at some point because they were stationed there or came home to look for work or be with family. But eight of them left again. For example, after retiring from the military, one tried to get a job in Hawai'i but was told "retired military are a dime a dozen here." So he extended his career with long-term jobs on the east and west coasts, finally retiring on the west coast. Another returned home after graduate school, but found "jobs were hard to come by." A third returned for a few years following a divorce, but left again with her second husband. Of the two interviewed in Hawai'i, one had returned after retirement to live in the family home; the other had returned to care for her aged father and was not sure if she would stay after he died, noting Hawai'i's limited work opportunities and low wages. All others planned to remain on the U.S. Continent, including nine with non-Hawaiian spouses, four with Native Hawaiian spouses, and three who were unmarried. The reasons for staying were summarized by a woman in Arizona who said:

> So after my husband died, I said, "you know, should I go back to Hawai'i?" You know, should I go ahead and go to Hawai'i or should I just stay here because my kids were here? And I decided to stay here. You know, all my kids are here and I have grand babies, and I have a house and friends, and it's affordable.

Advantages and disadvantages of living away from Hawai'i

When asked about advantages of living away from Hawai'i, 11 mentioned greater affordability and opportunities for home ownership. For example, one said "The expenses in Hawai'i are so high, and here you can buy a home, a very nice home, for probably half the cost of what you have to pay in Hawai'i." Another said, "I have classmates that never left Hawai'i, and even after retiring from a government job there, they never could actually own a house." Another said, "For me, it was pretty much based on finances. I just knew I could not afford to buy a home in Hawai'i."

Twelve mentioned better opportunities for work. For example, one participant said: "I became an aerospace engineer, and they didn't have jobs like that in Hawai'i." Another said, "Hawai'i gave me a hard time with my chiropractic license, so I moved to a state that accepted it, and I easily set up my practice." Others just liked the Continental U.S. ("I fell in love with San Francisco") or felt that Hawai'i was "just too small" after having lived a few years away.

Disadvantages included missing family (n = 10), Hawaiian food (n = 9), the 'āina (land) or environment (n = 10), the music (n = 10), and the aloha spirit (n = 12). The lack of aloha spirit was discussed in comments like "the Hawaiian aloha we miss, because people here are not as friendly as they are in Hawai'i" and "the aloha spirit is missing." A participant who moved back to Hawai'i to provide care to her father said:

The thing that the mainland does not have is our aloha spirit. And I still … although I certainly could be accused of being biased, feel like there is no kinder place that I've ever been to than Hawai'i. And so that is just something that I always missed, and I was always aware that I did not have that when I was living on the mainland.

Another explained:

I can remember walking down the road [on the Big Island] and people would say "hui! hele mai 'ai" (come in, come eat). And you go in to the kitchen of Tūtū (grandma), and all she'd have was a little bowl of beans and that was cooked in just salted water and a little bowl of poi (pounded taro), and she called you to have something to eat. You share. So when you grow up with that, with aloha, you share. And sometimes I look at people here who don't share, and I don't understand it, and I think "really?"

Another recounted:

I think particularly of Hilo [Hawai'i Island] where I was born and raised … As I was growing up and living there, there were a couple of very disastrous tsunami and very unexpected volcanic eruptions that, you know, turned people's lives upside down. But somehow people helped each other, and people recovered. And, so I think a lot of that spirit was instilled in me automatically as I was living there and growing up. There are nice people here, but it is not the same.

Another disadvantage was a feeling of disenfranchisement and loss. Four felt that, by living on the U.S. Continent, they were considered as "less Hawaiian" by their counterparts at home, and five felt that Hawai'i was "not the Hawai'i I left." One woman explained,

There is a fear of losing my 'Hawaiian-ness'. Sometimes, when I return home, I find that Hawaiian phrases and places have lost their significance. It takes me a week of just sitting and breathing in the Palolo [Valley] air to completely bring me home.

Racism as a push or pull factor

Unlike in our previous research (Browne & Braun, 2017), none of the participants reported racism as a push factor in leaving Hawai'i. However, in migrating to the U.S. Continent, 11 participants recounted direct experience with racism. For example, one participant, whose father was light skinned and whose mother was dark skinned, remembered having a hard time finding housing in California, hearing "oh, we don't rent to your kind." Two participants born in the Pacific Northwest were mistaken as American Indian or Hispanic and treated poorly. One explained, "Because Hawaiians look more like Indian, you know, you get treated more like Indian," while the other said "When you have a suntan, they expect that you are Hispanic, and you're supposed to speak Spanish. So I learned Spanish by osmosis and in self-defense." A male participant in the Western U.S. said:

We were very well aware of race because my wife is Caucasian. So my kids are hapa (mixed) … When we lived in the city and she'd be walking the kids, people assumed she was the au pair.

A woman who joined the Women's Army Corps and was sent for training in the U.S. South remembered:

I did not know whether I was black, white, or brown. I did not know which part of the bus to sit on. So, I sat in the middle, and I said I'd never go back down to Alabama again. So all the locals from Hawaiʻi, we just stayed on base.

Seven participants did not think they experienced racism directly. However, one recounted that her son experienced discrimination in Hawaiʻi when he attended a summer program for Hawaiian youth because, "he's very *haole* (Caucasian) looking." But she went on to say, "I never felt discrimination all the years living here on mainland." A participant who relocated as a child with her parents to Southern California explained:

[In Hawaiʻi] we went to Catholic School, so we didn't speak pidgin or anything so we didn't stand out. And in California, we went to another Catholic school. Other students were Guamanian, Mexican, Filipino, you know. So I didn't feel any big transition.

Another noted that the small size of his new town was an advantage in that he did not feel like a stranger for long, although some people called him by stereotyping nicknames:

[Where I lived] was a small town. So everybody knew everybody pretty much, you know. So when you went out, you ran into everybody, when they had parade and when I played softball. So you know, you go to the gym, you suddenly meet everybody. One of the company men for 5 years, he called me Pineapple and Coconut, and he asked me one day, 'What is your real name?'

Whether they personally experienced racism or not, eight said they were surprised either by the lack of minorities ("I'd look around, and I'd be the only person of color in the room") or the differential treatment of minorities after coming from a majority-minority state. A woman who attended college in the East said, "segregated housing was new to me." A woman who went to Chicago for college found:

Being a girl from Hawaiʻi made me very popular … But I could see right away that there were race differences you don't see in Hawaiʻi. I would see Black adults working at the fast-food places, where back home, this was a job the students did. It was really unusual to see someone making their living doing that. And the service industry was all African American, so it was a different experience, this racism.

Several found advantages to being Hawaiian. For example, one man said:

Even though I have some Hawaiian blood, I don't look very Hawaiian. So the only thing that set me apart was the name K. And you know, when I first got to

New York and I was looking for work, I would say, 'Gee, maybe I should become Jack or John or something people are more familiar with.' But I found that if you are looking for work in New York, and you have a name that nobody else has, that's an advantage because people will remember it.

Another participant noted advantages because of the timing of his migration, recounting:

When I moved to Washington, DC in the late 1960s and started work in 1970s, the Civil Rights laws and affirmative action programs were being implemented in the federal government (my employer for decades) to address racism in the workplace. I believe I benefited from them through increased opportunities for promotion. If I lived and worked in Hawai'i at that time, I don't believe the affirmative action programs would have been as beneficial to me.

Aging and caregiving

Participants related several ways that they cared for their aging parents. For the 14 whose parents lived in Hawai'i, two brought their parents to the U.S. Continent for care, three returned to Hawai'i to help provide care, and nine visited home to give respite to siblings providing care. In addition to helping care for parents, six cared for aged in-laws, five cared for disabled/dying spouses, two cared for disabled/dying friends, and one cared for a child who died in young adulthood.

While it is not possible to compare the rate of family caregiving between this group of Native Hawaiians and others, 15 respondents felt that Native Hawaiians, regardless of where they lived, were more likely than members of the dominant culture to care for their parents, saying "We don't call it a job ....we just take care of each other." As one man explained,

When you look at the caregiving, you have to look at it from a cultural perspective because culturally that's what the Hawaiians did, no matter who. I remember myself when I was a young one, they just take care of each other anyway they can. So you do the same thing. Not knowing that maybe long ago, unconsciously, these things were put in your mind. Because I never adjusted to more current thinking. The thought of putting my dad in the home never came to my mind ... just take care of him, that's all.

Three participants wondered if this would change with the increasing cost of living in Hawai'i and the continued migration of young Native Hawaiians to the U.S. Continent. A man in the Pacific Northwest explained:

You notice any of the neighbors in Hawai'i, you know, you see three generations under the same roof. A lot of it is economics. Nobody can afford a house, so rather than people moving out on their own, they stay. Here you could buy another house. Or if someone becomes of age, you could pack up and move them to an apartment because it's readily available and affordable. In Hawai'i, you can't afford to do that. They say, 'OK, let's just stay together in one place.'

When asked about their plans for their own aging, 16 felt they would stay on the U.S. Continent, desiring to age in place and/or move in with children and grandchildren. Seven said there were more eldercare resources on the U.S. Continent than in Hawai'i. Of the two who had returned to Hawai'i, one had the opportunity to age in place in the family home, but the other was unsure if she would stay after her parent's death, as the family house was to be sold and the proceeds distributed among the siblings. One man spoke of Native Hawaiian friends that returned to Hawai'i in retirement, saying:

> Some of them actually went home to finish, to live out their lives as opposed to staying up here. I don't know their cases. I don't know the driving force to go home. I guess all of us would love to be home. But for me that's not a [financial] reality of life.

Despite their preferred location for aging in place, 12 wanted to be buried or have their ashes scattered in Hawai'i. Of the six that did not, three were veterans who said they would be buried in a VA cemetery near their place of death.

Resilience and advice

Findings from this portion of the interview suggested that connections to family, other Hawaiians, and Hawaiian culture, along with financial well-being, contributed to the resilience of Native Hawaiians on the continent. The major areas of advice were to create new community wherever you go and to spread aloha.

All 18 recounted ways they kept in touch with the islands, family, other Hawaiian people, and Hawaiian food and culture. For example, 15 organized and/or attended regular reunions with family and high school classmates, as illustrated by one of the participants.

> We don't get home every year, but every year we go to Vegas. And the family from Hawai'i always comes up and so we'll meet. My wife comes from a family of 10 siblings, and so at any given time when you come to Vegas, going to be at least four or five of them that come up cuz they love to do their thing. Coming up there's a huge family reunion, because one of my wife's nephews is getting married in Vegas, so everybody's saving their money to be there. Even my two married sons and their kids are planning to go down and do this big thing with the family.

Seven participants specifically talked about how they accessed products from Hawai'i. A woman who started a hālau hula (hula school) said, "My mom would mail CDs for our club." A woman who wanted to introduce her babies to poi, the traditional first solid food of Hawaiian infants, said, "I was lucky because in Chicago there was a place I could buy frozen poi." A woman in Seattle said:

I miss Hawai'i and the sensations of Hawai'i. But every time I need a fix, I go to the Hawai'i General Store [in Seattle], smell the plumeria, the lei, and just pick up some dried crack seed. And the gal that owns it graduated from Punahou [High School], and the people that work there are from Hawai'i. So you know, they bring in lei, you can get poi every Thursday, you can get just about anything you want, just go down there. And there's plenty of Hawaiian contact.

Twelve participated in Hawaiian-oriented clubs, including local chapters of the Association of Hawaiian Civic Clubs, canoe clubs, hālau hula, and 50th State Clubs (these became popular after statehood in 1959). Fifteen found other Native Hawaiians living in their new communities. One woman told us, "I met my husband when we were in the service in Texas; he was from the Big Island." Another said, "I was impressed to see so many of us here, and many of them worked for the airlines."

These co-located Native Hawaiians came together to organize Hawaiian activities and clubs. For example, a man who met other Hawaiians stationed near him in Europe said, "So every place you go, you find the Hawaiians, and you associate with them to re-create what you left behind, you know, and you try to duplicate this." A woman in the Southwest said, "With so many, we have an annual Aloha Festival here. The hālau that come in are fabulous. We're spreading the aloha and it's great." A woman in Missouri said:

My friends and I just decided they wanted to get some exercise, so would get together and dance *hula*. It's just been a boost. It's something from my youth, and I love getting together to sing songs we haven't sung for 60 years. And now my granddaughter is learning the 'ukulele.

A woman in Arizona recounted:

We co-founded the first Hawaiian outrigger canoe club in the State of Arizona. And there's now four of them! We met L, and he owned the canoes, but he left them back in Santa Rosa. We said, 'Hey, the canoes are just sitting there, and nobody's using them. We're bringing them to Phoenix." So that's how we ended up founding it over here. So we paddled in the lakes. They even go compete. They go to the Lili'uokalani races. They have been to Brazil and Canada. They've been all over the place.

Another theme was financial stability, mentioned by nine participants. This included making a good salary during one's working years, and having a good retirement package with health insurance. One participant explained:

If you have a financial well-being, that allows you a lot more latitude. So fortunately I made some choice decisions early on. As a retired military person, I have the benefits of a military health program as well as a military pension. I had a very marketable degree and … . [after the military], I was able to parlay that into another job, and then another after that, so I earn pensions with both of those companies … I followed what my father and my uncle in Hawai'i had taught me was make sure you get your pensions, multiple pensions, so you can survive in retirement. Having that financial thing has helped us pay off the house here, and it's helped us to help the family members, my daughters and sons, so they could get themselves established.

When asked what advice they would give other Native Hawaiians migrating to the U.S. Continent, 17 said to "create community where you are." New community included family, other Native Hawaiians in the area, and non-Native Hawaiians with whom they shared interests. Eleven also would advise newcomers to remember their heritage, keep practicing it, and teach others about Hawaiian culture. A male participant, who reminded us that Hawaiians were voyagers and that Hawaiian chiefs had encouraged Hawaiians to go abroad, said:

> So if you leave an island in Hawai'i, you gotta bring that island with you here. And that means, the values and culture that you grew up with, the food stuffs that you need to live with, the music that you have. You bring your culture with you because your new island is going to be someplace else. So just like the Hōkūle'a [a contemporary Hawaiian voyaging canoe] had to take enough furnishings to live on the ocean, you got to take enough furnishings to live on another island.

A key component of this culture was most often referred to as the "aloha spirit," defined as "just caring and loving everybody" and "caring for yourself and your 'ohana (family)." Another explained how to manifest aloha spirit, saying, "I think, as long as you can help somebody out, you know, I think you should." A participant in the Pacific Northwest explained:

> Hawaiians are a unique people. I mean, no matter where we go, we're very well liked because we carry the culture. The aloha spirit carries real deep. It is the way that our parents raised us. It has to be felt, that's why. People who felt the aloha spirit, they go there, and they see the welcoming.

Some spoke to the spiritual aspects of "aloha spirit," saying, "no matter what you come into, just know that Akua (God) is going to be there, one way or another, whether you believe in him or not." Another said:

> For me again, advice for others is be who you are, be proud of who you are. And again, practice, practice aloha – you know, growing up there, we were aloha "Ke Akua (God) is love,' and treating everybody equally, fairly.

Six participants also spoke of a duty or strong desire to perpetuate the culture and to help other Native Hawaiians. For example, a woman in Texas said: "I pound my own poi here ... I give classes on that, and I give classes on how to make lei and hula skirts, and everybody has to make their own costumes." A group of Pacific Islanders on the West Coast decided to start a leadership training program for Pacific Islanders. A participant said:

> There's no other leadership course like it ... We instill in them the need to champion Pacific Islanders and give back to society ... One is now a legislator, one a professor, one opened a charter school in Utah, one is a social worker for Pacific Islander youth ... I'm so proud."

Another participant became a columnist for a Hawai'i-oriented newspaper:

> I would travel to different places in the Pacific Northwest to different Hawaiian events, and I did profiles on people from different areas and where they're from … So I met a ton of islanders who lived up here and I kind of did PR … Now, I say I'm an activist in the Hawaiian community – well actually the Pacific Islander community – to a point where a couple of years ago I was appointed to the university's minority advisory council. My activism has been to improve the situation for Pacific Islanders.

A woman from the Mid-West said:

> Because in Hawai'i you've got the Filipino, you got the Chinese, you've got the Thai and here, you have to kind of have to hunt around, you have to find out those different cultures, and learn to really appreciate the melting pot atmosphere that you have in Hawai'i that you can also have here. And identify for yourself what the aloha spirit is, what it means to feel a part of your community, to feel a part of your neighborhood and to share that.

Discussion

The stories of Native Hawaiian elders who have spent 30 or more years on the U.S. Continent are diverse and fascinating. Yet there were similarities across them. For the most part, they left for adventure and better work and educational opportunities, and they stayed because they built lives and community in their new homes. Most witnessed and/or experienced racism, but this did not prevent them from successfully negotiating their lives and developing networks to sustain and enrich them. Most cared for their aged parents, albeit most did it from afar and in support of siblings providing direct care in Hawai'i. All were proud of their Hawaiian heritage, and most were actively practicing and supporting Hawaiian cultural activities in their new communities. All felt that a strength of the Hawaiian culture was the aloha spirit, defined as caring for others and treating others as equals, and most advised other Hawaiians living abroad to live this value.

The Native Hawaiians interviewed in this study appear to be similar to people of other ethnic groups who move from one U.S. state to another (Frey, 2009). Americans migrate across states for work or education or to follow parents and partners. They enter new communities and make new friends. When they meet others from their own culture and/or hometown, they may feel more cultural ease to befriend them, especially if this can involve the sharing of foods, music, dialect, and other familiarities of home. If racism is encountered, migrants may have fewer options for socialization, further encouraging them to cluster together, which may further reinforce cultural traditions (Browne & Braun, 2017; Meyer, 2003). In the case of our participants, however, all expanded their networks to non-

Hawaiians in their new communities and freely shared information and practices from the islands, thus "spreading aloha."

Several important Hawaiian values should work against migration for Native Hawaiians. One is a strong "sense of place." From cultural anthropology and geography, locations with a strong sense of place have a strong identity that is deeply felt by inhabitants and visitors (Relph, 2008). In Hawai'i, sense of place often manifests as a sense of reverence for and familiarity with a specific part of the islands or feelings of belongingness and well-being associated with a specific community or ahupua'a or the 'āina in general. This sense of place was reflected in the fondness with which participants spoke of their ancestral homes, and many recounted lessons and values they carried with them from those places. Despite living away for 30 or more years and having plans to age in place and die on the U.S. Continent, fully two-thirds wanted to be buried or to have their ashes spread in Hawai'i. This suggests that place continues to be important to Native Hawaiians that leave Hawai'i.

Besides a sense of place, an important Hawaiian value is kuleana, which is most commonly translated as responsibility, privilege, authority, or concern associated with being part of the larger social fabric of the family and community (Ewalt & Mokuau, 1995). In traditional culture, different members of the family (and the community) had specific kuleana. Having someone in the family migrate may leave these roles unfilled or require others to take them on. Although we did not ask about kuleana in a systematic way, conversation revealed that most of our participants had siblings who stayed behind to carry out family-related duties, which eventually encompassed elder care. Many participants, even those not involved in daily eldercare, expressed a clear kuleana for family to care for elders. Also, most mentioned that they were encouraged or supported by family to leave (at least temporarily). In fact, only one participant said that his parents did not want him to move away, and another mentioned that his family eventually adopted someone from outside the family to fulfill the duties our participant left behind.

Thus, for our participants (and the parents of the participants who grew up on the Continent), their initial moves are explained by the pull of adventure and better school and work opportunities, combined with the push of Hawai'i's high cost of living, the support of parents, and the presence of siblings who would fulfill family care obligations in their absence. All of our participants then found the means (e.g., parental support, scholarships, military, savings) to leave Hawai'i.

Although racism was not a push factor for migration for our participants, once on the Continent, 13 participants witnessed and/or directly experienced racism, and five did not. Variation in experiences with racism was likely due to a number of factors. Skin tone was mentioned by several kūpuna, with more negative experiences for those with darker skin and more positive experiences for those with lighter skin. Phenotype discrimination (or discrimination based on an overt characteristic such as skin color) has long been a part of U.S. culture and has been linked to reduced opportunities for economic and social advancement and to poor health outcomes (Jones et al., 2008; Wilson et al., 2010).

Location and timing also were factors. For example, those who migrated to Southern California reported less discrimination than those who went to the U.S. South. The two who went to primary and secondary school in rural areas in the Pacific Northwest recounted direct experiences of discrimination, whereas others who migrated as adults to larger cities in the Pacific Northwest did not. Migrating pre- vs. post-statehood (1959) may also have made a difference. After statehood, the nation started to become more curious about Hawaiʻi, and the islands became a romantic and desirable tourist destination (not without its own problems of commodification and exotifcation of Hawaiian culture and people).

We were somewhat surprised that racism in Hawaiʻi was not mentioned as a push factor. This is something we heard from a number of participants in earlier qualitative research with Native Hawaiians who had migrated to Southern California (Browne & Braun, 2017). This is perhaps partially explained by the timing of migration. Although we did not systematically ask for the year of migration, Native Hawaiians in our first research cohort were older than participants in the current study. Many left the islands prior to the resurgence of Hawaiian pride in the 1970s (termed the Hawaiian Renaissance) that ultimately led to constitutional amendments that made Hawaiian an official language of the state, established the Office of Hawaiian Affairs, supported Hawaiian education in schools, and laid the groundwork for the return of the island of Kahoʻolawe, used by the US military for bombing practice for decades, and the protection of the customary rights of Native Hawaiians (Marsella et al., 1995). Those who left prior to the Hawaiian Renaissance may have encountered more interpersonal bias and structural racism than those who left later, and were thus pleasantly surprised by the opportunities open to them in Southern California. Future research in this area should more systematically track timing of migration and other variables that may help explain the variation in experiences of racism.

Several resilience factors were identified, including staying in touch with Hawaiian family and values, financial security, and a passion to promote aloha. The leading pieces of advice were to create community where you are and to perpetuate the aloha spirit. Research on the aloha spirit is limited, but a cross-sectional survey of 1,028 undergraduates at the University of Hawaiʻi found that students in high agreement with this statement "Have you learned the Aloha Spirit in Hawaiʻi?" reported significantly lower levels of psychological distress and a reduced risk of depression, even after controlling for self-reported discrimination, race/ethnicity, immigrant status, duration of residence in Hawaiʻi, and other factors (Mossakowski & Wongkaren, 2016). Among these students, Native Hawaiians scored the highest (3.8 out of 4), while Whites scored the lowest (3.0 out of 4). These findings lend support to the notion that the aloha spirit, however defined, is an important resilience factor for Hawaiians at home and abroad.

Limitations

The study has several limitations. First, we did not interview participants in all 50 states. Second, research participants are volunteers, and findings could be subject to volunteer bias, i.e., healthier and better educated individuals are more likely to participate in research than those with fewer assets (Ganguli et al., 1998). In fact, 40% of our participants reported their health as excellent or very good, compared to only 29% of Native Hawaiians age 60+ in Hawaiʻi, and none of our respondents reported their health as poor, compared to 18% within the state (Hawaiʻi State Department of Health, 2019). Furthermore, 61% of our participants had a baccalaureate degree or higher, compared to 14% of Native Hawaiians in the state (Hawaiʻi State Department of Business and Economic Development, 2016). Third, our study did not gather similar data from a sample of kūpuna who never left Hawaiʻi, which would have been useful for comparison. However, in 2018, Kamehameha Schools began a study of Native Hawaiians who had moved away, those who moved away and returned to Hawaiʻi, and those that never left.

Implications for social work practice and policy

Social workers need to know that Native Hawaiian elders, regardless of where they are living, strive to retain their culture, maintain a strong "a sense of place," and honor kuleana in their caring for family and kūpuna. Findings also lend support to previous research that Native Hawaiians on the Continent may be "healthier and wealthier" than those in Hawaiʻi (Nakatsuka et al., 2013). Further quantitative research is needed to examine health and socioeconomic differences in kūpuna living on the Continent vs. Hawaiʻi.

Earlier studies on the health and long_term service and support (LTSS) needs and care preferences of Native Hawaiian elders in Hawaiʻi identified inadequate finances and a preference for culturally anchored programs and providers (Browne et al., 2014). In this present study, the financial need of Native Hawaiians on the U.S. Continent was less emphasized and subsequently, there was less discussion around housing and financial assistance supports such as SSI and Medicaid assistance – lifeline programs for those living in or near poverty. Moreover, our study participants could not name any specific aging program or service, with some commenting that the

Continental U.S. appeared to have more services and options for older adults than did Hawaiʻi. Programs funded through Title VI of the Older Americans Act are in alignment with national directions to help elders age in place (Browne et al., 2015), but elders and families need to know more about these and other services.

Social and health care interventions anchored in Native Hawaiian cultural values have shown positive improvements in health outcomes and service utilization in Hawaiʻi (Braun et al., 2014; Kaʻopua et al., 2011; Mokuau et al., 2012). Similar studies have not been conducted on the continent. In the absence of any clear data on care preferences, it may be helpful for aging and LTSS providers to focus on improving service information and accessibility, and to target Native Hawaiians "where they gather," for example, through Civic Clubs, high school reunions, and cultural groups and festivals.

Policy-level interventions should promote healthy aging and reduce health disparities, i.e., those differences in health that are "unnecessary, avoidable, unfair and unjust, and warrant remedial action" (Sadana et al., 2016, p. S179). Although the focus of this study was not on Native Hawaiians in Hawaiʻi, our results point to multilevel factors that contribute to differences in healthy aging across these two geographical contexts. If Native Hawaiians on the U.S. Continent prove to be "healthier and wealthier" compared to those residing in Hawaiʻi, additional study will help to uncover and understand the reasons for this disparity. It may well be that policies and interventions in Hawaiʻi need a continued and greater emphasis on the social determinants of health, including income, housing, education, working conditions, and discrimination.

In addition to disparities, we believe it is also important that studies such as ours document and acknowledge the resiliencies and strengths in a population. We heard from our participants less of a need for financial assistance and more about the strength found in maintaining a strong sense of community with other Native Hawaiians and Hawaiian culture. Examples of resilience-promoting strategies included interventions that promote healthy family relations, financial security, and social connections through Hawaiian cultural opportunities. More robust studies should examine healthy aging from an equity perspective to understand the broader determinants of healthy aging and the role of culture and geography in meeting LTSS needs.

Finally, as noted earlier, much of our knowledge base about Native Hawaiians comes from data collected on the Hawaiian archipelago. However, with increasing cost of living in Hawaiʻi and continued emigration of young people, we can project that the Native Hawaiians will be increasingly scattered across the globe. Vigorous comparative data will help to tease out the health profiles of those on the U.S. Continent and Hawaiʻi and, subsequently, the practice and policy approaches that should be targeted to improve the health of both groups. Given national and global trends in migration, social workers will continue to be challenged to develop an improved understanding of human movement within and across borders and how best to advocate and serve. In the end, actions that improve socio-economic conditions and enforce anti-discriminatory measures will likely offer the best hope for a healthy aging for all people.

Conclusion

In summary, we used focused ethnography to interview 18 Native Hawaiian elders who lived away from Hawai'i for 30+ years. In general, they found greater opportunities for education, work, and home ownership, and did not lose their deep connection to their culture, to the aloha spirit, and to Hawai'i as a geographic and spiritual home.

Acknowledgments

We gratefully acknowledge the support of our elder study participants. We also thank the members of our Joint Advisory Council, composed of the Native Advisory Council and the Partner Organizations: Dr. Kūhiō Asam, Ms. Nalei Akina, Ms. Caroline Cadirao, Dr. J. Keawe'aimoku Kaholokula, Dr. Shawn Malia Kana'iaupuni, Sister Alicia Damien Lau, Dr. Diane Paloma, Ms. Deborah Stone Walls, Ms. Kealoha Takahashi, Ms. Leslie Tanoue, and Dr. Lisa Watkins-Victorino.

Disclosure statement

No potential conflict of interest was reported by the authors.

Funding

This project was supported, in part, by the US Administration on Aging, Department of Health and Human Services, Washington, D.C. 20201 by grant number to Hā Kūpuna National Resource Center for Native Hawaiian Elders [90OI0007/01]. Grantees undertaking projects under government sponsorship are encouraged to express freely their findings and conclusions. Points of view or opinions do not, therefore, necessarily represent official government policy.

ORCID

Kathryn L. Braun ⓘ http://orcid.org/0000-0002-1586-0252
Rachel Burrage ⓘ http://orcid.org/0000-0003-0143-1147
Yan Yan Wu ⓘ http://orcid.org/0000-0003-1553-1392

References

Brandolo, E., Gallo, L. C., & Meyers, H. F. (2009). Race, racism, and health: Disparities, mechanisms, and interventions. *Journal of Behavioral Medicine, 32*(1), 1–8. https://doi.org/10.1007/s10865-008-9190-3

Braun, K. L., Browne, C., Ka'opua, L. S., Kim, B. J., & Mokuau, N. (2014). Research on indigenous elders: From positivistic to decolonizing methodologies. *The Gerontologist, 54*(1), 117–126. https://doi.org/10.1093/geront/gnt067

Braveheart, M. Y., & Debruyn, L. M. (1998). The American Indian holocaust: Healing historical unresolved grief. *American Indian and Alaska Native Mental Health Research, 8* (2), 56–78. Retrieved from http://europepmc.org/abstract/MED/9842066

Browne, C., & Braun, K. L. (2017). Away from the islands: The diaspora's effects on Native Hawaiian elders and families in California. *Journal of Cross-cultural Gerontology, 32(4),* 395–411. https://doi.org/10.1007/s10823-017-9335-3

Browne, C., Carter, P., & Gray, J. (2015). National resource centers focus on indigenous elder communities. *Generations, 38*(4), 70–73. https://search.proquest.com/openview/107d953f2800f389cfa9d771308112b8/1?pq-origsite=gscholar&cbl=30306

Browne, C., Mokuau, N., & Braun, K. L. (2009). Adversity and resiliency and adversity in the lives of Native Hawaiian elders. *Social Work, 54(3),* 253–261. https://doi.org/10.1093/sw/54.3.253

Browne, C., Mokuau, N., Ka'opua, L. S., Kim, B. J., Higuchi, P., & Braun, K. L. (2014). Listening to the voices of Native Hawaiian elders and 'ohana caregivers: Discussions on aging, health and care preferences. *Journal of Cross Cultural Gerontology, 29*(2), 131–151. https://doi.org/10.1007/s10823-014-9227-8

Creswell, J. W., & Poth, C. N. (2018). *Qualitative inquiry and research design: Choosing among five traditions.* Sage Publications.

Ewalt, P., & Mokuau, N. (1995). Self-determination from a Pacific perspective. *Social Work, 40*(2), 168–175. https://doi.org/10.1093/sw/40.2.168

Frey, W. H. (2009). *The great American migration slowdown: Regional and metropolitan dimensions.* Metropolitan Policy Program at the Brookings Institution. Retrieved from https://www.brookings.edu/wp-content/uploads/2016/06/1209_migration_frey.pdf

Ganguli, M., Lytle, M. E., Reynolds, M. D., & Dodge, H. H. (1998). Random versus volunteer selection for a community-based study. *Journals of Gerontology: Medical Sciences, 53*(1), M39–46. https://doi.org/10.1093/gerona/53a.1.m39

Goodyear-Ka'opua, N., Hussey, I., & Wright, E. K. A. (2014). *A nation rising: Hawaiian movements for life, land, and sovereignty.* Duke University Press.

Hausmann, L. R. M., Kressin, N. R., Hanusa, B. H., & Ibrahim, S. A. (2010). Perceived discrimination in health care and its association with patient's healthcare experiences: Does the measure matter? *Ethnicity & Disease, 20* (1), 40–47. Retrieved from https://www.ethndis.org/priorarchives/ethn-20-01-40.pdf

Hawai'i State Department of Business and Economic Development. (2016, January). *Educational attainment in Hawai'i. Statistical brief, January 2016.* Hawai'i State Department of Business and Economic Development. Retrieved from http://files.hawaii.gov/dbedt/economic/data_reports/briefs/Educational%20Attainment_Jan_2016.pdf)

Hawai'i State Department of Health. (2019). *Self-rated health by age and ethnicity (2011–2016).* Honolulu, HI: Hawai'i State Department of Health. Retrieved from http://ibis.hhdw.org/ibisph-view/query/result/brfss/GenHealth4Cat/GenHealth4CatCrude11_.html

Jones, C. P., Truman, B. I., Elam-Evans, L. D., Jones, C. A., Jones, C. Y., Jiles, R., & Perry, G. S. (2008). Using "socially assigned race" to probe white advantages in health status. *Ethnicity & Disease*, *18* (4), 496–504. Retrieved from https://www.ethndis.org/priorarchives/ethn-18-04-496.pdf

Ka'opua, L. S., Park, S. H., Ward, M., & Braun, K. L. (2011). Testing the feasibility of a culturally tailored breast cancer screening intervention with native Hawaiian women in rural churches. *Health & Social Work*, *36*(1), 55–65. https://doi.org/10.1093/hsw/36.1.55

Kaholokula, J. K. (2014). Achieving social and health equity in Hawai'i. In J. N. Goodyear-Ka'opua & A. Yamashiro (Eds.), *The value of Hawai'i 2: Ancestral roots, Oceanic visions* (pp. 254–264). University of Hawai'i Press. https://doi.org/10.13140/2.1.4188.7522

Kirmayer, L. J., Tait, C. L., & Simpson, C. (2000, September). The mental health of Aboriginal peoples in Canada: Transformations of identity and community. *Canadian Journal of Psychiatry*, *45*(7), 607–616. https://doi.org/10.1177/070674370004500702

Marsella, A. J., Oliveira, J. M., Plummer, C. M., & Crabbe, K. M. (1995). Native Hawaiian culture, mind and well-being. In H. I. McCubbin, E. A. Thompson, A. I. Thompson, & J. E. Fromer (Eds.), *Resiliency in ethnic minority families* (pp. 93–113). University of Wisconsin.

Mayan, M. J. (2009). *Essentials of qualitative inquiry.* Routledge-Taylor and Francis.

Merry, S. E. (2000). *Colonizing Hawai'i: The cultural power of law.* Princeton University Press.

Meyer, I. H. (2003). Prejudice, social stress, and mental health in lesbian, gay and bisexual populations. Conceptual issues and research evidence. *Psychological Bulletin*, *129*(5), 674–697. https://doi.org/10.1037/0033-2909.129.5.674

Mokuau, N., Braun, K. L., & Daniggelis, E. (2012). Building family capacity for Native Hawaiian women with breast cancer. *Health & Social Work*, *37*(4), 216–224. https://doi.org/10.1093/hsw/hls033

Mokuau, N., Browne, C., Braun, K. L., & Choy, L. (2008). Using a community-based participatory approach to create a resource center for Native Hawaiian elders. *Health for Education*, *21* (3), 174–178. Retrieved from https://www.ncbi.nlm.nih.gov/pubmed/19967637

Mossakowski, K. N., & Wongkaren, T. S. (2016). The paradox of discrimination, the "aloha spirit," and symptoms of depression in Hawai'i. *Hawai'i Journal of Medicine and Public Health*, *75* (1), 8–12. Retrieved from https://www.ncbi.nlm.nih.gov/pmc/articles/PMC4733820/pdf/hjmph7501_0008.pdf

Nakatsuka, N. J., Esquivel, L. M., Levin, M. J., Browne, C. V., & Braun, K. L. (2013). Identifying the unique challenges facing Kanaka Maoli *kūpuna* residing outside of Hawai'i. *Hūlili*, *9(1)*, 133–151. Retrieved from http://www.kamehamehapublishing.org/hulili_9/

O'Brien, B. C., Harris, I. B., Beckman, T. J., Reed, D. A., & Cook, D. A. (2014). Standards for reporting qualitative research: A synthesis of recommendations. *Academic Medicine*, *89*(9), 1245–1251. https://doi.org/10.1097/ACM.0000000000000388

Pearlin, L. I., Schieman, S., Fazio, E. M., & Meersman, S. C. (2005). Stress, health, and the life course: Some conceptual perspectives. *Journal of Health and Social Behavior*, *46*(2), 205–219. https://doi.org/10.1177/002214650504600206

Piché, V. (2013). Contemporary migration theories as reflected in their founding texts. *Population*, *68* (1), 141–164. Retrieved from https://www.cairn-int.info/article-E_POPU_1301_0153-contemporary-migration-theories-as-refle.htm

Relph, E. (2008). *Place and placelessness.* Sage Publications.

Sadana, R., Blas, E., Budhwani, M. A., Koller, T., & Paraje, G. (2016). Healthy ageing: Raising awareness of inequities, determinants, and what could be done to improve health equity. *The Gerontologist*, *56*(S2), S178–193. https://doi.org/10.1093/geront/gnw034

Siriwardhana, C., Ali, S. S., Roberts, B., & Stewart, R. (2014). A systematic review of resilience and mental health outcomes of conflict-driven adult forced migrants. *Conflict and Health*, *8*(13). https://doi.org/10.1186/1752-1505-8-13

Sotero, M. M. (2006). A conceptual modal of historical trauma: Implications for public health practice and research. *Journal of Health Disparities Research and Practice*, *1* (1), 93–108. Retrieved from https://papers.ssrn.com/sol3/papers.cfm?abstract_id=1350062

Stanley, L., Swaim, C. R., Kaholokula, J., Kelly, K., Belcourt, A., & Allen, J. (2017). The imperative for research to promote health equity in Indigenous communities. *Prevention Science*, 2020;21(Suppl 1):13-21. https://doi.org/10.1007/s11121-017-0850-9

Sue, D. W., Capodilupo, C. M., Torino, G. C., Bucceri, J. M., Holder, A. M. B., Nadal, K. L., & Esquilin, M. (2007). Racial microaggressions in everyday life: Implications for clinical practice. *American Psychologist*, *62*(4), 271–286. https://doi.org/10.1037/0003-066X.62.4.271

U.S. Census. (2012). *The Native Hawaiian and other Pacific Islander population: 2010*. U.S. Department of Commerce. Retrieved from https://www.census.gov/newsroom/blogs/random-samplings/2012/06/2010-census-shows-native-hawaiians-and-other-pacific-islanders-surpassed-one-million.html

Wainberg, M. L., Alfredo González, M., McKinnon, K., Elkington, K. S., Pinto, D., Gruber Mann, C., & Mattos, P. E. (2007). Targeted ethnography as a critical step to inform cultural adaptations of HIV prevention interventions for adults with severe mental illness. *Social Sciences and Medicine*, *65*(2), 296–308. https://doi.org/10.1016/j.socscimed.2007.03.020

Wilson, K. B., Hinojosa, T. J., & Gines, J. G. (2010). Phenotype discrimination: Outcomes based on race, disability status and gender in the United States. In J. A. Jaworski (Ed.), *Advances in Sociology Research* (pp. 175–191). Nova Science Publishers, Inc.

Wu, Y. Y., Braun, K. L., Horiuchi, B. Y., Tottori, C., Wilkens, L., & Onaka, A. T. (2017). Life expectancies in Hawai'i: A multi-ethnic analysis of 2010 life tables. *Hawai'i Journal of Medicine and Public Health*, *76(1)*, 9–14. Retrieved from https://www.ncbi.nlm.nih.gov/pmc/articles/PMC5226016/

Part 2

Promising Interventions for Indigenous Health Equity

"Togetherness:" the role of intergenerational and cultural engagement in urban American Indian and Alaskan Native youth suicide prevention

Celina M. Doria, Sandra L. Momper, and Rachel L. Burrage (iD)

ABSTRACT

In a collaborative study with an Urban Indian Health Organization (UIHO) and a University, we conducted six talking circles over three years with American Indian and Alaskan Native (AI/AN) elders, adults, and youth to examine perceptions of suicide and suicide prevention strategies within their community. Results of a thematic analysis indicated that normalization of suicide, stigma, and historical trauma were barriers to suicide prevention. Consistent themes of elders, adults, and youth over all three years reflected the need for intergenerational engagement and cultural connectedness as suicide prevention strategies. Implications for culturally-grounded social work practice with AI/ANs are presented.

Background

Suicide rates within American Indian and Alaskan Native (AI/AN) populations are among the highest in the United States, with rates being 3.5 times higher than other racial and ethnic groups (Leavitt et al., 2018). Suicide is the leading cause of death for youth aged 10–24 (Centers for Disease Control and Prevention, 2015), and AI/AN youth are at disproportionately higher risk (National Institute of Mental Health, 2015). According to the Michigan Department of Health and Human Services (MDHHS), AI/ANs in Southeast Michigan (where this study occurred) experience higher suicide death rates than other populations (Michigan Department of Health and Human Services, 2016). In 2015, the reported rates of suicide deaths in Michigan per 100,000 people for AI/ANs was 26.5, compared to 14.3 for Whites and 5.8 for Blacks (Michigan Department of Health and Human Services, 2016). The rates of suicide deaths for youth aged 10–24 were similarly high, with 11.4/100,000 AI/AN youth dying by suicide, compared to 9.7 Whites and 7.1 Blacks (Michigan Department of Health and Human

Services, 2016). Given these numbers, suicide prevention has emerged as a critical response to this public health crisis.

Suicide risk factors

Substance use

AI/AN youth are disproportionately vulnerable to substance use which increases the likelihood of suicide attempts and completions (Beals et al., 2005; Dickerson & Johnson, 2012). In 2013, it was reported that AI/AN youth had the highest lifetime prevalence of substance use, with 39% of youth aged 12 to 17 reporting illicit drug use (Substance Abuse and Mental Health Services Administration, 2014). Alcohol use and binge drinking – both related to suicide attempts and deaths among AI/ANs – disproportionately impact AI/ANs, as they have the highest prevalence of a positive family history for alcoholism of all ethnic groups in the United States (Barlow et al., 2012).

Health, mental health, and trauma

Decreased health and mental health status of AI/ANs is often attributed to impacts of historical trauma, loss of identity, and lack of social support (Barlow et al., 2012; Gone, 2013). Historical trauma is defined as psychological and emotional "wounding" occurring due to an experience of collective trauma (Brave Heart et al., 2011, p. 283). Experiences of land dispossession, forced relocation and removal, exploitation, and racism, coupled with persisting state-sponsored violence, have resulted in extreme poverty rates, heightened health disparities, and increased instances of substance abuse (Brave Heart et al., 2011; Brown et al., 2016). The mental well-being of AI/ANs is further diminished by the internal conflict of walking in two worlds – or living between traditional ways and the dominant culture's ways (Brown et al., 2016). These compounding experiences of historical and interpersonal traumas place AI/AN youth at increased risk to die by suicide.

Limited access to, and cultural appropriateness of, mental health care

These risk factors are amplified by limited access to – and underutilization of – mental health services, reducing help seeking behaviors among AI/AN youth (Hartmann & Gone, 2013). Access is especially limited for urban AI/ANs. The 2010 U.S. Census reports that 78% of the 5.2 million AI/ANs live in urban areas, yet less than 1% of Indian Health Services (IHS) funds are allocated to urban centers (U.S. Department of Health and Human Services, 2017).

A contributing factor to the underutilization of mental health services relates to the discord between traditional healing practices and Western psychotherapy models. Lack of cultural competency among White therapists and Western therapy models that do not consider AI/AN worldviews perpetuate underutilization (Hartmann & Gone, 2013). Mistrust in the mental health system and other federal institutions – due to traumatic histories – negatively impacts service utilization (Freedenthal & Stiffman, 2007). Nationally, AI/AN users of community mental health services make up only 0.5% of consumers (Substance Abuse and Mental Health Services Administration, 2017). However, AI/ANs in the Midwest have the greatest penetration of mental health service use compared to other minority groups (Substance Abuse and Mental Health Services Administration, 2017). Consequently, there is a greater need for behavioral health providers that are culturally competent and accepting of blending traditional practice with that of Western practice. The fragmentation and lack of cultural connection for urban AI/AN communities contributes to diminished help seeking, ultimately contributing to increased rates of suicide (Weaver, 2012).

Protective factors against suicide

Cultural and community connectedness
Previous research indicates that prevention strategies that involve community and family participation in collectively creating culturally-grounded interventions, coupled with an awareness of historical trauma, can best promote AI/AN youths' wellness (Brave Heart et al., 2011; Wexler et al., 2015). While much literature focuses on the vulnerabilities and risk factors of AI/AN youth, it is important to recognize the unique strengths and protective factors specific to AI/AN youth, which include cultural values and community connectedness (Burrage et al., 2016; McMahon & Kenyon, 2013). Traditional knowledges, cultural practices, and community and family connectedness, have been cited as protective factors against suicide (DeCou et al., 2013; Stiffman et al., 2007). Family, generosity and helping, spirituality, and respect for elders are all essential values held by AI/ANs (House et al., 2006) and a family's relationship with elders has been linked to increased resilience (Johnson, 1995). A focus on the unique values and strengths of AI/AN communities presents a more holistic and strength-based perspective of Native well-being and creates space to consider culturally-relevant suicide prevention strategies.

Purpose of the present study

This study expands upon previous literature by highlighting the important role of cultural and community connectedness in AI/AN suicide prevention. The focal research questions were: 1) How much does the local community know about AI/AN youth suicide prevention efforts at the UIHO? 2) What are the community's perceptions of the strengths and weaknesses of the AI/AN youth suicide prevention efforts at the UIHO? and 3) What are the community's suggestions for improving AI/AN youth suicide prevention efforts at the UIHO? By attending to the community's culturally-grounded perceptions of suicide prevention strategies and support, this study attempts to fill the dearth of research examining ways to improve help seeking strategies among AI/AN elders, adults and youth, in their own words.

Methods

Setting

The study took place at a large Midwestern Urban Indian Health Organization (UIHO), which serves AI/AN people from a seven-county area, as well as those who are not AI/AN. The 2010 U.S. Census reports that 48,000 people who identify as AI/AN, or AI/AN and another race, reside in this area (U.S. Census Bureau, 2010) The UIHO incorporates Western health models and traditional AI/AN healing to empower individuals and families to enrich their physical, mental, spiritual, and emotional well-being. The center has over 40 staff and also utilizes volunteers and interns from local universities. It holds community events including an annual powwow, winter solstice, sweat lodges, and naming ceremonies. Since 2011, the UIHO has received SAMHSA funding to conduct suicide prevention and intervention activities to include focus groups conducted as talking circles, gatekeeper trainings, suicide screenings, educational interventions, and wellness activities. Recent community suicide screenings with the youth (ages 10–24) revealed that 10% of the youth had *attempted* suicide in the past, all but one of whom were AI/AN (Mueller-Williams, Tauiliili, Momper, Tuomi, & Bieber, 2015).

Research approach

This study used data from six Community Readiness Assessment (CRA) focus groups. The CRA framework is a community-based participatory research (CBPR) approach designed to engage local community members in the development of intervention strategies to address a specific issue (Israel et al., 1998; Jumper-Thurman et al., 2003; Minkler & Wallerstein, 2008). This model catalyzes a community's readiness to act to address an issue by increasing knowledge and awareness, promoting local leadership, and utilizing local resources to support change efforts (Jumper-Thurman et al., 2003). The CRA framework also promotes a high level of community ownership, values their specialized knowledge and commitment to addressing identified issues, and creates space for sustainable change.

The CRA focus groups were adapted to be conducted like talking circles (not a *sacred* talking circle), which are a traditional method of group communication in AI/AN communities. Other AI researchers have successfully used talking circles, as the circles rely on oral tradition to relay experiences (Becker et al., 2006; Hodge et al., 2002). Community members and the research team adapted the CRA interview protocol for use in these talking circles. Purposive sampling was utilized to capitalize on local knowledge and expertise. Agency staff and community members (elders, adults, youth) who frequented the UIHO were invited – via face-to-face and telephone contact – to participate in the talking circles.

All researchers had some prior connection to the UIHO. The second author moderated the talking circles, is American Indian, and has worked with the UIHO on a number of research projects. The first and third authors have both previously completed clinical internships with the UIHO. Consequently, the research team was familiar with the UIHO, its services, and the local community context to the project.

Measures

The talking circles utilized a protocol of 10 questions that were both open-ended (i.e. "What do you know about suicide prevention at the Indian center?") and closed-ended (i.e. "How many people are aware of the National Suicide Prevention hotline?") to provide participants an opportunity to respond as they felt comfortable. A demographic survey and Likert scale survey measuring participants' experiences with suicide were also used. The demographic survey included 20 questions regarding tribal affiliation, gender and sexual identity, living situation, education level, employment status, and household income. It also included two questions regarding whether or not the participant knew anyone who had "attempted" or "died by suicide." The Likert scale survey included 5 questions using a scale from 1–10 (with 1 being "not at all" and 10 being "a very great concern"). An example question included: "how much of a concern is AI/AN youth suicide in the community?"

Procedure

The CRA talking circles were conducted at the UIHO with elders and adults (ages 18 and older) in March 2015, May 2016, and May 2017. Separate CRA talking circles were conducted with youth (ages 7 to 17) in May 2015, June 2016, and April 2017. Informed consent/assent was received from participants for both the talking circle and the audio recording; those participants under age 18 had parent/caregiver consent. Prior to beginning, a meal was provided and the group smudged. Smudging involves the group standing in a circle and burning sage in a shell as a form of cleansing; the shell is passed around and people are cleansed by the smoke, and then an elder or leader says a brief prayer for a good meeting. Participants sat in a circle and everyone had equal opportunity to speak. The talking circles lasted approximately one hour. Participants were compensated with a 20 USD gift card.

Data analysis

The CRA talking circles were recorded and transcribed by the first author. The transcriptions were read and a thematic analysis was completed following Braun and Clarke (2006) *15- Point Checklist of Criteria for Good Thematic Analysis*. The thematic analysis was inductive, limiting the data to what was explicitly stated by the participants to ensure the data were participant-driven (Braun & Clarke, 2006). The data were open-coded to identify quotes and excerpts of text that illuminated the identified themes and sub-themes. Themes that were not related to resources and challenges of suicide prevention were excluded from the final thematic structure. The coded data were reviewed and re-coded by the first author to ensure the fidelity of the identified themes, resulting in six revisions to the thematic structure. Each of the various codes were then grouped into three overarching themes and made into visual representations that the first author presented to the second and third authors for suggestions and revisions. Demographic survey results were entered into SPSS for analysis of frequencies and descriptives. We do not report on the Likert survey results here. The UIHO approved this study and the University's Institutional Review Board deemed this study to be exempt as all data were de-identified.

Results

Participant characteristics

There were 6–16 participants per talking circle, with the majority of participants self-identifying as AI/AN or AI/AN and one or more other race. The six focus groups were comprised of 32 youth, and 44 elders/adults. They ranged in age from 7 to 83; 34 identified as male, 37 as female, and 2 as two-spirit (see Table 1). Notably, the majority of the youth participants identified as more than one race, while the majority of the elder and adult participants identified as AI/AN. Participants reported knowing 49 people who had attempted suicide and 39 who had died by suicide. Most participants had some form of suicide prevention training (e.g., safeTALK and Applied Suicide Intervention Skills Training) in which they acquired skills at recognizing and referring someone at risk of suicide for an intervention

Table 1. Demographic characteristics of talking circle participants.

Characteristics	Youth Participants 2015		Youth Participants 2016		Youth Participants 2017		Adult/Elder Participants 2015		Adult/Elder Participants 2016		Adult/Elder Participants 2017	
Total Participants	16		10		6		14		14		16	
Gender												
Female	6	37.5%	5	50%	3	50%	7	50%	8	57%	8	50%
Male	8	50%	5	50%	3	50%	7	50%	5	36%	6	37.5%
Two-Spirit											2	12.5%
No answer	2	12.5%							1	7%		
Age												
8– 13 Years	9	56%	2	20%	3	50%						
14– 17 Years	4	25%	8	80%	3	50%						
18– 24 Years							1	7%	2	15%	2	12.5%
25– 34 Years							1	7%			1	6.25%
35– 44 Years							1	7%	3	21%	1	6.25%
45– 54 Years							3	21%	3	21%	3	18.75%
55+ Years							6	43%	5	36%	6	37.5%
No answer	3	19%					2	15%	1	7%	3	18.75%
Race and Ethnicity												
Native American, American Indian, Alaskan Native/ First Nations	1	6.25%					8	58%	11	79%	12	75%
Native Hawaiian or other Pacific Islander	1	6.25%										
Hispanic or Latino	1	6.25%	2	20%	2	33%					1	6.25%
Asian							1	7%				
Black or African American							1	7%				
Caucasian/White							2	14%				
Arab American												
AI/AN and one or more other race	11	68.75%	8	80%	4	67%	2	14%	3	21%	3	18.75%
No answer	2	12.5%										
Suicide Prevention Trainings Attended												
0	6	37.5%	5	50%	4	67%	6	43%	7	50%	7	43.75%
1– 3	7	43.75%	2	20%	2	33%	7	50%	6	43%	6	37.5%
4– 7			3	30%			1	7%			2	12.5%
8– 10									1	7%	1	6.25%
10+												
No answer	3	18.75%										
Suicide History												
Someone you know has attempted suicide.	4	25%	2	20%					4	29%	3	18.75%
Someone you know has died by suicide.					1	17%	2	14.5%	1	7%	1	6.25%
Both of the above.	2	12.5%	5	50%	1	17%	10	71%	7	50%	11	68.75%
None of the above.	6	37.5%	3	30%	4	66%	2	14.5%	2	14%	1	6.25%
No answer.	4	25%										

(LivingWorks, 2018). The majority were involved members of the UIHO, including members of the youth group and community advisory council.

Themes

Three themes were identified for both the youth and the elder/adult talking circles. The youth participants discussed theme 1) the duality of suicide: normalization and stigmatization, theme 2) becoming a source of knowledge to prevent suicide, and theme 3) intergenerational engagement as prevention strategy. The elders and adults discussed theme 1) historical trauma as a barrier to help seeking, theme 2) connecting to culture to prevent suicide, and theme 3) and intergenerational engagement as prevention strategy. Intergenerational engagement was a consistent theme over all three years and was overlapped between both youth and elders/adults.

Youth talking circles
Theme one: the duality of suicide: normalization and stigmatization. Youth from all three talking circles identified conflicting, sometimes ambivalent feelings about suicide in their community. Many reported feeling that suicide is both normalized and stigmatized within the community. This dual understanding of suicide created a barrier to help seeking as the youth felt both accustomed to suicide and ashamed of talking about it.
Normalization of suicide. Given the high frequency of completed suicides among AI/AN youth, suicide became something to be expected within their community. Many shared that while suicide was commonplace in their community, there was a lack of acknowledgment of the problem:

Participant 1: I think since suicide happens so much in the communities, people just take it as a normal thing.

Participant 2: Because it's happening so frequently these days, a lot of people are just in denial that it even happens.

Participant 3: Everyone knows it's there because it's so prevalent in the community [...] So everyone knows it's there, everyone sees it, [but] not everyone talks about it.

Another participant expressed how the normalization of suicide influences the underutilization of prevention services:

> People have grown accustomed to it. They're like 'Oh that happened. It's sad.' And I think that the other problem is that people are either too scared to talk about it or kinda just brush it off their shoulder like 'oh, that's not gonna happen to anyone in my family or my friends.'

Many felt that the normalization of suicide decreased the likelihood that people would disclose feelings of suicidality. One youth shared that suicide is viewed as "one of those don't ask, don't tell situations," highlighting the secrecy and silence about suicide within the community. Through its normalization, suicide was seen as a less important issue among the youth, resulting in a cycle of silence, underutilization of services, and high death rates. Increasing outreach and awareness of suicide in the community – particularly within local schools – was cited by many youth as a way to decrease the normalization of suicide and increase help seeking behaviors.

Stigmatization of suicide. The majority of the youth participants discussed the stigma that surrounds mental health and suicide within the community. One of the youth participants explained how stigma inhibits prevention and contributes to the underutilization of mental health services:

> One of the barriers is fear [because] a lot of people are scared to talk about or learn about suicide or suicide prevention. It's like a touchy thing […] so a lot of people don't really wanna address it, but that's holding a lot of people back. [I]f you're too scared to learn about it, or talk about it, or address it to somebody then you're not helping anyone.

Many identified the negative perceptions of suicide held among the community. Said one participant: "I think that people feel disgusted that somebody wants to end their life." One youth frankly stated that suicide is "a stupid thing." This stigma – the feelings of fear, disgust, stupidity – that surrounds suicide decreased the likelihood that the youth would report feelings of suicidality, as they were "scared to talk about it." Feeling marked by this stigma, some youth felt that lack of trust among social and familial networks contributed to underreporting of suicidality and underutilization of support services.

Theme two: becoming a source of knowledge to prevent suicide. Improved capacity building as a result of increased knowledge of suicide prevention was cited as a facilitator of help seeking. Many of the youth participants recognized the relevance of their knowledge and expertise as a way to increase suicide prevention. As one youth suggested, "Sometimes *we* can be a source of information cuz we can tell our family and sometimes they can tell other friends." The youth felt more capable of supporting their community by increasing their knowledge of suicide and suicide prevention strategies. One participant identified how an increased knowledge of suicide can affect the larger community: "You don't feel like you're alone and that, that's part of suicide prevention too, it's us, togetherness." Another youth suggested, "We become sources for people to talk to us about it." This increased awareness of suicide prevention strategies encouraged and empowered the youth to assist their community members in need.

Participating in suicide trainings at the UIHO and other activities was integral in increasing youth knowledge and capacity. As one participant shared, "some of us in this talking circle do use some of the skills we're taught to prevent suicide." One youth participant explained, "before I had the training and I didn't really know what to do. Now I do feel a bit more prepared, but I also feel more aware of the warning signs and seeing things more from a preventative place." Increased capacity and knowledge empowered the youth to both provide prevention efforts and seek support when needed. Each youth participant could identify sources of support in help seeking, including talking with the staff of the UIHO, school counselors, family members, and peers.

While the majority of the youth felt empowered to "talk" about suicide, others felt the individual burden of preventing suicide was overwhelming. One participant shared: "I'd like to think I'd be able to [support a suicidal friend or family member], but I don't necessarily know if I'd be able to handle it myself or not." Being the keepers of this knowledge led some youth to feel overwhelmed by the perceived responsibility to "act" when confronted by a suicidal community member. One participant explained: "I feel like it's extremely scary. Like what if you say something that triggers them." Despite these fears, the majority of the youth felt more capable of preventing suicide in their community as they gained more knowledge.

Theme three: intergenerational engagement as prevention strategy. Many of the youth participants cited the lack of community, due to an "age divide" between the youth and adults, as an obstacle to suicide prevention. This segregation between age groups hindered help seeking, as some youth mentioned feeling isolated and afraid to talk to others. One participant explained: "Some kids might not think that the adults understand like what they're going through or like they have no one to talk to who they trust, or are just like afraid to open up." Intergenerational engagement was not limited to connection with elders and adults. Many of the youth suggested integrating younger children into suicide prevention education and training. Said one participant:

> I feel like maybe we should have the little kids come in once in a while, because we do spend time together and they do see us as role models or older brothers and sisters, regardless of if we're related or not. And little kids don't really confide in parents and grown-ups; they come to their big brothers and sisters, [...] so being able to let them know that you're here for them, while talking about this topic, would make them not feel so uncomfortable about it. Like we'll do this together.

According to one participant, integrating the age groups would help "build a healthy community, like a big family, so people don't feel so alone. They could see themselves belonging in the community. They get a sense of purpose; see they have a place where they belong."

Many participants cited the positive impact familial relationships had on decreasing suicidality and increasing help seeking. One youth shared their personal story: "I used to go to this school and everyone just bullied me there, and one time I just had enough, so I wanted to commit suicide, but my brother told me not to." Additionally, the majority of the participants cited their parents and other adult figures as people whom they would talk to if they were feeling down, depressed or suicidal. Thus, strengthening the intergenerational engagement and support between elders/adults and youth served as a positive protective factor against suicide.

Adult talking circles

Theme one: historical trauma as a barrier to help seeking. The collective history of trauma that AI/AN populations have experienced was identified and discussed by the adult participants in all three talking circles, revealing the connection between historical trauma and suicide. One participant synthesized the impact of historical trauma on the present-day community:

> I look at the big picture, the pressures, that particularly come out in Indigenous people but the genocidal practices have … taken away their roles, and stopped them, and killed them, and made them … a life where they can't see what's worth living – putting up with this pain.

Many participants cited forced removals and experiences of boarding schools as traumatic events that have continued to affect the community today. One participant candidly proclaimed: "I think [the high suicide rate] is about the boarding schools." As suggested by the adults, previous trauma has a large impact upon the lived experiences of the AI/AN populations, illuminating their perceptions and understandings of suicide.

Theme two: connecting to culture to prevent suicide. Preserving cultural traditions was the most salient recurring theme that arose from all three adult talking circles. Many participants spoke to the importance of preserving their traditions and upholding their cultural values as a means to prevent suicide. As one participant shared, "we are competing with mainstream society when it comes to our way of life." Multiple participants identified feeling "frustrated" by Western mental health services, and identified a need to incorporate traditional healing practices, including talking circles, into mental health practices to promote help seeking behaviors. Working with a "Native healer" or "spiritual advisor" were suggested to support wellness. For many, the UIHO successfully integrated traditional practices that promote cultural preservation. One participant shared: "Being Native American would have been misunderstood [had I sought services elsewhere]." Another participant shared the impact of these talking circles on her healing:

[O]ne of the things that I found comforting for myself, as well in the suicide prevention efforts, was that the talking circles existed. Several of us have already brought up being able to bring one's challenges out [to] the community [during these talking circles]. It not only destigmatizes [suicide], but it humanizes what you experience, because you are able to learn from others.

Another participant explained the necessity of preserving cultural practices: "Because when you are living in a bigger environment that has its goal to destroy [AI/AN] identity then it's seen as more important to put that element in there and to fight for that." Through a process of preserving cultural practices, participants felt they could maintain their identity. For the adult participants, this is a vital means of suicide prevention.

Cultural teachings were identified as an important aspect of suicide prevention. One participant noticed during their experience of volunteering with the youth that "there is a lack of understanding of the importance of cultural preservation." Another participant explained: "It's teaching, uh, you know, your culture, teaching the culture, and getting them involved early, you know teaching them how to drum and sing and things like that and be more involved with each other as a family." Many of the adult participants believed that by valuing cultural teachings and creating a sense of community, mental health and well-being would be greatly improved.

Theme three: intergenerational engagement as prevention strategy. Increasing mutual support and "intergenerational connection" among elders, adults, and youth was identified as an important protective factor to prevent suicide. One participant expressed "there are no roles for young warriors anymore," which they felt led to a lack of cultural identity and influenced suicide risk. Many participants discussed early intervention strategies – including increased outreach by adults in elementary school settings – in order for "the kids to know that they aren't alone, however they feel." Increased need for parental engagement was a recurring theme identified by the group. The participants suggested that an increased involvement of parents would increase their capacity to prevent suicide among the youth. One participant explained: "You gotta remember there are parents going through the same things that the youth are going through. And kids don't talk to their parents, they talk to the leaders in the program instead of us." By increasing parental engagement in suicide prevention efforts, participants suggested they would be better able to support their children and strengthen the whole community.

Discussion

The elders, adults and youth identified important themes regarding suicide risk and strategies for suicide prevention. While the youth participants emphasized normalization and stigmatization of suicide as risk factors, the elders and adults stressed the role of historical and intergenerational trauma in contributing to the high rates of suicide within the community. Youth stressed becoming knowledgeable about suicide to prevent suicide, and both groups suggested an increase in intergenerational engagement, while at the same time highlighting the role of community connectedness and cultural knowledge as a protective factor.

Urban AI/AN youth face challenges as they navigate their mental wellness and cultural identity. Many urban AI/AN youth feel isolated from their culture and racially marginalized, resulting in greater feelings of isolation, sadness, and suicidal ideation (Weaver, 2012). These environmental factors reinforce the paradoxical understanding of suicide – normalization and stigmatization – identified by the youth from the talking circles (Binnix et al., 2017). When suicide is both expected and feared, AI/AN youth experiencing suicidal ideation must choose between silence, being stigmatized for disclosing their feelings, or death by suicide. This tension generates a vicious cycle of silence, stigmatization, and suicide, compromising youths' mental well-being, inhibiting help seeking, and perpetuating high rates of suicide within the community. While other studies have explored the effects of vicious cycles of silence and stigma (Beadle-Holder, 2011; Binnix et al., 2017; Harris et al., 2011), there is a dearth of research on this topic in regards to AI/AN youth suicide. As the elders, adults, and youth in this study expressed, this cycle of silence, stigmatization, and suicide can be prevented by increasing the connection to culture and community. Traditional knowledge and cultural values – passed down by elders and adults – can help to break the silence and prevent suicide. The results of this study have practical implications for suicide prevention in AI/AN communities.

This study highlights the important role of cultural and community connectedness to prevent youth suicide. Prior research with AI/ANs has cited connectedness as a culturally based protective factor against suicide (Mohatt et al., 2011). Other studies have shown that resilience among AI/AN communities is gained through connection to culture and community (Browne et al., 2009; Hill, 2009; Kahn et al., 2016; Schultz et al., 2016). For the participants in this study, cultural connectedness represented knowledge of cultural teachings and practices (e.g., drumming), and preservation of cultural knowledge, while community connectedness represented intergenerational relationship-building and engagement. While culture and community are distinct concepts, each offering unique strategies for suicide prevention, they are intimately tied together within Indigenous worldviews. Connectedness represents the spiritual interweaving of family, community, land, animals, ancestors, and traditional knowledges (Hill, 2009). Together, increasing cultural and community connectedness may generate a greater sense of belonging, identity, and purpose among AI/AN youth, ultimately fostering resilience and protecting against suicide.

As this study shows, intergenerational engagement, coupled with traditional knowledge, can act as an intervention strategy to increase connection to both culture and community. As described by the study participants, cultural connection is passed down through AI/AN elders, who are recognized as the keepers and disseminators of knowledge and ways of life for their communities. The way in which they engage with youth can have profound impacts on the well-being of the community at large (Kahn et al., 2016). Intergenerational relationships foster protection against suicide by increasing community connectedness and support, positively influencing help seeking and resilience (DeCou et al., 2013). Engagement among different age groups increases connection to culture as elders are able to pass down traditional knowledge and cultural values (Kahn et al., 2016). As our study shows, elders are willing to engage in cultural teachings with the youth to strengthen their connection to culture, ultimately reinforcing the sense of community. The findings of this study suggest that connectedness to culture and community, supported by intergenerational engagement, has the potential to increase suicide prevention among AI/AN youth.

The methodology of the talking circles utilized in this study may function as a dual research intervention and suicide prevention method. While some literature suggests talking circles are successful in implementing health behavior change programs with AI/AN communities (Gone, 2013; Mehl-Madrona, 2014), there is limited research related to utilizing talking circles as both research and prevention method for examining AI/AN youth suicide. Talking circles are culturally grounded, utilizing oral history traditions to tell stories and relay information (Becker et al., 2006). Having culturally relevant care available to the AI/AN community increases the likelihood of help seeking and service utilization, contributing to lower rates of suicide (Gone, 2013; Hartmann & Gone, 2013; US. Department of Health and Human Services, 2010). Talking circles also represent a community-based, collaborative research method that can promote sustained solutions to suicide prevention. This dual intervention highlights a community-based response to this public health crisis.

Limitations and future research

The specific location of the study makes the results ungeneralizable to all AI/AN populations, as it is important to remember the great diversity among AI/AN communities across the U.S. The number of participants in this study were small as is common in focus groups. Also, we utilized purposive sampling techniques in order to ensure some homogeneity in each talking circle and reach elders, adults, and youth.

While challenges and supports to help seeking and suicide prevention strategies were derived from this data, there may be additional challenges or resources not mentioned. Future studies might include intergenerational focus groups/talking circles in which the themes of this study were further explored and possible solutions, or avenues for implementation, are shared between the age groups. Despite these limitations, few such stories exist on AI/AN views on suicide and this presents an opportunity to share their knowledge.

Implications for social work practice

Findings from this study contribute to the knowledge base on suicide intervention and prevention among AI/AN populations from the perspectives of elders, adults, and youth. The themes highlight the need for social workers to be culturally aware of the perceptions of suicide and means of prevention that urban AI/AN populations embrace. Results indicate that there is an increase in community awareness and an emphasis on traditional cultural practices as healing. Overall, it is clear that through an increased knowledge of suicide and prevention strategies, the stigma surrounding suicide is decreased, though it persists. This study highlights talking circles as an effective, culturally-grounded method of suicide prevention and research intervention. By bringing together elders, adults, and youth, the community is able to share collective knowledge and traditions, strengthen cultural ties, and increase resilience. Most notably, our study reinforces the role of cultural and community connectedness in suicide prevention for AI/AN individuals and families. This study ultimately uplifts the voices of urban AI/AN elders, adults, and youth, as they put forth their own recommendations and strategies toward preventing suicide within their community.

Maamwimaashkogaabawiying: Together we are Strong and Still Standing.

Acknowledgments

Miigwetch, thank you, to community member participants and this UIHO's Suicide Prevention Team. This study is funded by the Substance Abuse and Mental Health Services Administration Garrett Lee Smith State and Tribal Youth Suicide Prevention Grant #U79 SM061738-01. The views, opinions, and content does not necessarily reflect the views, opinions, or policies of the Center for Mental Health Services, SAMHSA, or the U.S. Department of Health and Human Services.

Disclosure statement

No potential conflict of interest was reported by the authors.

Funding

This work was supported by the Center for Mental Health Services [U79 SM061738-01].

ORCID

Rachel L. Burrage ⓘ http://orcid.org/0000-0003-0143-1147

References

Barlow, A., Tingey, L., Cwik, M., Goklish, N., Alchesay, M., Lee, A., & Strom, R. (2012). Exploring binge drinking and drug use among American Indians: Data from adolescent focus groups. *The American Journal of Drug and Alcohol Abuse, 38*(5), 409–415. https://doi.org/10.3109/00952990.2012.705204

Beadle-Holder, M. (2011). Black churches creating safe spaces to combat silence and stigma related to AIDS. *Journal of African American Studies, 15*(2), 248–267. https://doi.org/10.1007/s12111-011-9159-0

Beals, J., Novins, D., Whitsell, N., Spicer, P., Mitchell, C., & Manson, S. (2005). Prevalence of mental disorders and utilization of mental health services in two reservation populations: Mental health disparities in a national context. *American Journal of Psychiatry, 162*(9), 1723–1732. https://doi.org/10.1176/aapi.ajp.162.9.1723

Becker, S. A., Affonso, D. D., & Blue Horse, B. M. (2006). Talking circles: Northern Plains tribes American Indian women's views of cancer as a health issue. *Public Health Nursing, 23*(1), 27–36. https://doi.org/10.1111/j.0737-1209.2006.230105.x

Binnix, T. M., Rambo, C., Abrutyn, S., & Mueller, A. S. (2017). The dialectics of stigma, silence and misunderstanding in suicidality survival narratives. *Deviant Behavior, 39*(8), 1095–1106. https://doi.org/10.1080/01639625.2017.1399753

Braun, V., & Clarke, V. (2006). Using thematic analysis in psychology. *Qualitative Research in Psychology, 19* (2), 77–101. Retrieved from http://eprints.uwe.ac.uk/11735.

Brave Heart, M., Chase, J., Elkins, J., & Altschul, D. (2011). Historical trauma among Indigenous peoples of the Americas: Concepts, research, and clinical considerations. *Journal of Psychoactive Drugs, 43*(4), 282–290. https://doi.org/10.1080/02791072.2011.628913

Brown, R., Dickerson, D., & D'Amico, E. J. (2016). Cultural identity among urban American Indian/Alaskan Native youth: Implications for alcohol and drug use. *Prevention Science, 17* (7), 852–861. https://doi.org/10.1007/s11121-016-0680-1

Browne, C., Mokuau, N., & Braun, K. (2009). Adversity and resiliency in the lives of Native Hawaiian elders. *Social Work, 54*(3), 253–261. https://doi.org/10.1093/sw/54.3.253

Burrage, R. L., Gone, J. P., & Momper, S. L. (2016). Urban American Indian community perspectives on resources and challenges for youth suicide prevention. *American Journal of Community Psychology, 58*(1–2), 136–149. https://doi.org/10.1002/ajcp.12080

Centers for Disease Control and Prevention. (2015). *10 leading causes of death by age group, United States – 2015*. Centers for Disease Control and Prevention. Retrieved from https://webappa.cdc.gov/sasweb/ncipc/leadcause.html

DeCou, C., Skewes, M., & López, E. (2013). Traditional living and cultural ways as protective factors against suicide: Perceptions of Alaska Native University students. *International Journal of Circumpolar Health, 72*, 1–5. https://doi.org/10.3402/ijch.v72i0.20968

Dickerson, D., & Johnson, C. (2012). Mental health and substance abuse characteristics among a clinical sample of urban American Indian/Alaskan Native youths in a large California metropolitan area: A descriptive study. *Community Mental Health Journal, 48* (1), 56–62. https://doi.org/10.1007/s10597-010-9368-3

Freedenthal, S., & Stiffman, A. (2007). "They might think I was crazy:" Young American Indian's reasons for not seeking help when suicidal. *Journal of Adolescent Research*, *22*(1), 58–77. https://doi.org/10.1177/0743558406295969

Gone, J. P. (2013). Redressing First Nations historical trauma: Theorizing mechanisms for indigenous culture as mental health treatment. *Transcultural Psychology*, *50*(5), 683–706. https://doi.org/10.1177/1363461513487669

Harris, L. H., Debbink, M., Martin, L., & Hassinger, J. (2011). Dynamics of stigma in abortion work: Findings from a pilot study of the Providers Share Workshop. *Social Science & Medicine*, *73*(7), 1062–1070. https://doi.org/10.1016/j.socscimed.2011.07.004

Hartmann, W., & Gone, J. (2013). American Indian and Alaskan Native mental health. In M. Shally-Jensen (Ed.), *Mental health care issues in America: An encyclopedia* (pp. 40-47). ABC-CLIO, LLC.

Hill, D. L. (2009). Relationship between sense of belonging as connectedness and suicide in American Indians. *Archives of Psychiatric Nursing*, *23*(1), 65–74. https://doi.org/10.1016/j.apnu.2008.03.003

Hodge, F. S., Pasqua, A., Marquez, C. A., & Geishirt-Cantrell, B. (2002). Utilizing traditional storytelling to promote wellness in American Indian communities. *Journal of Transcultural Nursing*, *13* (1), 6–11. Retrieved from http://www.ncbi.nlm.nih.gov/pmc/articles/PMC3098048/.

House, L. E., Stiffman, A. R., & Brown, E. (2006). Unraveling cultural threads: A qualitative study of culture and ethnic identity among urban Southwestern American Indian youth, parents and elders. *Journal of Child and Family Studies*, *14*(4), 393–407. https://doi.org/10.1007/s10826-006-9038-9

Israel, B. A., Schulz, A. J., Parker, E. A., & Becker, A. B. (1998). Review of community-based research: Assessing partnership approaches to improve public health. *Annual Review of Public Health*, *19*(1), 173–202. https://doi.org/10.1146/annurev.publhealth.19.1.173

Johnson, A. F. (1995). Resiliency mechanisms in culturally diverse families. *The Family Journal: Counseling and Therapy for Couples and Families*, *3*(4), 316–324. https://doi.org/10.1177/1066480795034005

Jumper-Thurman, P., Edwards, R., Plested, B., & Oetting, E. (2003). Honoring the differences: Using community readiness to create culturally valid community interventions. In G. Bernal, J. Trimble, K. Burlew, & F. Leung (Eds.), *Handbook of racial & ethnic minority psychology* (pp. 591–607). Sage Publications.

Kahn, C. B., Reinschmidt, K., Teufel-Shone, N. I., Oré, C. E., Henson, M., & Attakai, A. (2016). American Indian elders' resilience: Sources of strength for building a healthy future for youth. *American Indian and Alaska Native Mental Health Research (Online)*, *23*(3), 117–133. https://doi.org/10.5820/aian.2303.2016.117

Leavitt, R. A., Ertl, A., Sheats, K., Petrosky, E., Ivey-Stephenson, A., & Fowler, K. A. (2018). Suicides among American Indian/Alaska Natives — National violent death reporting system, 18 states, 2003–2014. *Morbidity and Mortality Weekly Report 2018*, *67*, 237–242. https://doi.org/10.15585/mmwr.mm6708a1

LivingWorks. (2018). LivingWorks. Retrieved from https://www.livingworks.net/programs/

McMahon, T., & Kenyon, D. (2013). "My culture, my family, my school, me:" Identifying strengths and challenges in the lives and communities of American Indian youth. *Journal of Child and Family Studies*, *22*(1), 694–706. https://doi.org/10.1007/s10826-012-9623-z

Mehl-Madrona, L. (2014). Introducing healing circles and talking circles into primary care. *The Permanente Journal*, *18*(2), 4–9. https://doi.org/10.7812/TPP/13-104

Michigan Department of Health and Human Services. (2016). *Source: Division for Vital Records and Health Statistics. Report requested by AIHFS for specific Native American*

Raw Data. Michigan Department of Health and Human Services. Retrieved from https:// www.michigan.gov/mdhhs/0,5885,7-339-73970_2944_4669_4686—,00.html

Minkler, M., & Wallerstein, N. (Eds.). (2008). *Community based participatory research for health: From process to outcomes.* John Wiley & Sons, Publishers.

Mohatt, N. V., Fok, C. C. T., Burket, R., Henry, D., & Allen, J. (2011). Assessment of awareness of connectedness as a culturally-based protective factor for Alaska native youth. *Cultural Diversity & Ethnic Minority Psychology, 17*(4), 444–455. https://doi.org/ 10.1037/a0025456

Mueller-Williams, A.M., Tauiliili, D., Momper, S.L., Tuomi, A., & Bieber, C. (2015). "I'm grateful for waking up every morning:" Screening for suicide risk among American Indian/Alaska Native and First Nations youth. [Conference session]. American Public Health Association 2015 Annual Meeting, Chicago, IL, United States.

National Institute of Mental Health. (2015). *Suicide. National Institutes of Health.* National Institute of Mental Health. Retrieved from https://www.nimh.nih.gov/health/statistics/sui cide/index.shtml

Schultz, K., Sabina, C., Jackson, S., Cattaneo, L., Brunner, L., & Serrata, J. (2016). Key roles of community connectedness in healing from trauma. *Psychology of Violence, 6*(1), 42–48. https://doi.org/10.1037/vio0000025

Stiffman, A., Brown, E., Freedenthal, S., House, L., Ostmann, E., & Yu, M. S. (2007). American Indian youth: Personal, familial and environmental strengths. *Journal of Child and Family Studies, 16*(1), 331–346. https://doi.org/10.1007/s10826-006-9098-y

Substance Abuse and Mental Health Services Administration. (2014). *Results from the 2013 National survey on drug use and health summary of National findings,* NSDUH Series H-48, HHS Publication No. (SMA) 14-4863. Retrieved from https://www.samhsa.gov/data/ sites/default/files/NSDUHresultsPDFWHTML2013/Web/NSDUHresults2013.pdf

Substance Abuse and Mental Health Services Administration. (2017). *Michigan 2017 mental health National Outcome Measures (NOMS): SAMHSA uniform reporting system.* Substance Abuse and Mental Health Services Administration. Retrieved from https://www.samhsa. gov/data/report/2017-uniform-reporting-system-urs-table-michigan

U.S. Census Bureau. (2010). *American fact finder.* [Data file]. U.S. Census Bureau. Retrieved from https://factfinder.census.gov/faces/nav/jsf/pages/index.xhtml

U.S. Department of Health and Human Services. (2017). *Indian health service office of urban Indian health programs strategic plan 2017–2021.* U.S. Department of Health and Human Services. Retrieved from https://www.ihs.gov/urban/includes/themes/newihstheme/display_ objects/documents/IndianHealthServiceOfficeofUrbanIndianHealthProgramsStrategicPlan. pdf

US. Department of Health and Human Services. (2010). *To live to see the great day that dawns: Preventing suicide by American Indian and Alaskan Native youth and young adults.* DHHS Publication SMA (10)-4480, CMHS-NSPL-0196. Retrieved from https://www.sprc. org/sites/default/files/migrate/library/Suicide_Prevention_Guide.pdf

Weaver, H. (2012). Urban and Indigenous: The challenges of being Native American in the city. *Journal of Community Practice, 20*(4), 470–488. https://doi.org/10.1080/10705422. 2012.732001

Wexler, L., Chandler, M., Gone, J., Cwik, M., Kirmayer, L., LaFromboise, T., Brockie, T., O'Keefe, V., Walkup, J., & Allen, J. (2015). Advancing suicide prevention research with rural American Indian and Alaskan Native populations. *American Journal of Public Health, 105*(5), 891–899. https://doi.org/10.2105/AJPH.2014.302517

"Being on the walk put it somewhere in my body": The meaning of place in health for Indigenous women

Angela R. Fernandez ⓘ, Tessa Evans-Campbell, Michelle Johnson-Jennings, Ramona E. Beltrán, Katie Schultz, Sandra Stroud, and Karina L. Walters

ABSTRACT

Relationship to place is integral to Indigenous health. A qualitative, secondary phenomenological analysis of in-depth interviews with four non-Choctaw Indigenous women participating in an outdoor, experiential tribally specific Choctaw health leadership study uncovered culturally grounded narratives using thematic analysis as an analytic approach. Results revealed that physically being in historical trauma sites of other Indigenous groups involved a multi-faceted process that facilitated embodied stress by connecting participants with their own historical and contemporary traumas. Participants also experienced embodied resilience through connectedness to place and collective resistance. Implications point to the role of place in developing collective resistance and resilience through culturally and methodologically innovative approaches.

Introduction

Indigenous peoples' relationship to place is a critical component of health and well-being (Walters, Beltrán et al., 2011). The ongoing loss and destruction of land, along with limited access to healthy environments (Lewis et al., 2017) have been a major contributor to stress and negative health outcomes that reflect substantial health disparities between Indigenous and settler colonial populations (Hoover et al., 2012; Walters, Beltrán et al., 2011). A recent review of health intervention literature among Indigenous peoples of North America revealed the limited attention given to the role of connection to place in Indigenous health (Fernandez, 2019). The purpose of this study is to explore how physically walking parts of the Choctaw Trail of Tears in an experiential, place-based pilot study, impacted non-Choctaw Indigenous women's (NCIW) views on stress and resilience.

Indigenous health is conceptualized holistically across spiritual, emotional, mental, and physical domains and encompassed within familial, communal, and natural environment relationships (Vukic et al., 2011). The natural or physical environment is a core protective factor and an important determinant of health and wellbeing, which must be considered in improving Indigenous health (Jennings et al., 2018). Extending beyond land-based, geographic sites, Indigenous notions of place can also be socially constructed (Ramirez, 2007) wherein narratives of both trauma and healing can aid in prevention efforts (Fernandez, 2019). Further, places in which historical trauma events occurred may invoke both positive and negative feelings, as places hold memories of the past that are essential to framing historical and contemporary understandings (Dodge, 2007).

Historical trauma (HT) refers to cumulative and pervasive intergenerational trauma that arises as an outcome of human-made traumatic events targeting a specific community (Sotero, 2006; Walters, Mohammed et al., 2011), and the aftermath from historically traumatic events is at the root of settler colonial disruptions of Indigenous peoples' social, cultural, corporeal, and terrestrial relationships with the land in the United States (e.g., Walters, Beltrán et al., 2011; Walters & Simoni, 2002). Historical trauma events (HTE) are systematic attempts to destroy spiritual, cultural, and subsistence practices often based on relationships with land (Brave Heart et al., 2011; Evans-Campbell & Walters, 2006), thereby eliminating some of the core protective factors foundational to Indigenous health, and increasing vulnerability to stress and illness. Examples include restrictions on Indigenous agricultural methods and land use, land confiscation, and forced displacement imposed through federal policies (Calloway, 2008), which were designed to increase the environmental dispossession of Indigenous people from their lands through limiting access to traditional environments (Richmond & Ross, 2009). Effects of these assaults persist through ongoing environmental hazards related to for-profit initiatives such as the construction of pipelines and mining projects which threaten tribal sacred sites and water safety (e.g., Hoover et al., 2012; Lewis et al., 2017; Willox et al., 2013).

The contemporary health sequelae of such HTE among Indigenous peoples are evident in their significant health disparities compared to non-Indigenous groups. Resulting disparate health outcomes include alarming rates of obesity, diabetes, and heart disease, associated with food insecurity among tribal communities in North America (First Nations Development Institute, 2013). Additionally, climate change – largely the result of human activity – is dramatically reducing sea ice, thereby limiting Arctic Indigenous peoples' subsistence practices, leading to increased reports of anxiety and depression, and a decreased sense of health and well-being overall (Willox et al., 2013). Such impacts of environmental change on marginalized

Indigenous communities increase vulnerability to poor health and mental health outcomes (Billiot et al., 2019).

Stress and resilience related to Indigenous relationships to place can be embodied. Embodiment refers to how societal and ecological circumstances become biologically incorporated and can manifest in health outcomes across generations (Krieger, 2005). Indigenous scholars have incorporated this concept into their framing of the relationship between place and health (Beltrán et al., 2018; Schultz et al., 2016). Indigenous peoples' concept of connectedness, defined as "the interrelated welfare of the individual, one's family, one's community, and the natural environment" (Mohatt et al., 2011, p. 444), provides a culturally specific context in which these embodied relationships can be understood. Importantly, place-related stress can manifest in the embodiment of both the memory and contemporary manifestations of HTE. This embodied stress, coupled with a reduction in protective factors, results in negative, intergenerational health consequences (Krieger & Davey Smith, 2004; Walters, Mohammed et al., 2011). For example, Indigenous peoples today across tribal nations experience loss and grief surrounding widely shared historical trauma events such as displacement or boarding school abuses, even if they or their ancestors did not directly experience these traumas (Whitbeck et al., 2004).

Despite hundreds of years of settler colonial attempts to sever Indigenous relationships to place, Indigenous bodies, minds, and spirits continue to be sites of resilience. Indigenous resilience is a multi-level, evolving, transformative, and adaptive social and psychological process, characterized by positive outcomes at the personal, familial, community and larger social group levels (Kirmayer et al., 2011). Simultaneously, Indigenous peoples' resistance is a crucial part of their resilience. The opposition of oppression through actively upholding Indigenous identities, lifeways, and ontologies can be viewed as coping mechanisms (e.g., Alfred & Corntassel, 2005). Such coping mechanisms can be reinforced within relationships between strong families and communities, and with language, storytelling, spirituality, and engaging with the land through cultural, spiritual, and subsistence practices (Alfred & Corntassel, 2005). These efforts can also be conceptualized as "survivance," which emphasizes Indigenous peoples' active presence (including ties to homelands) through continuation of stories that renounce Indigenous erasure and victimization (Vizenor, 2008).

Over the past several decades, Indigenous scholars have contributed to the ongoing work of communities and practitioners to transform the adverse impacts of historical trauma through innovative theory, research, and interventions. Indeed, research on the role of place and settings in Indigenous health interventions is steadily growing (Beltrán et al., 2018; Fernandez, 2019; Jennings et al., 2018; Schultz et al., 2016; Walters, Beltrán et al., 2011). One widely used model, the Indigenist stress-coping model (ISCM; Walters &

Simoni, 2002), posits that cultural and spiritual buffers moderate the relationship between traumatic stressors and poor health outcomes in Indigenous populations. Within the ISCM, the Indigenous connection to place is an integral context and consequence of events and activities in both the "trauma" domain (e.g., historical trauma via displacement) and the "cultural buffers" domain (e.g., traditional health practices) identified in the model. This informs our proposed conceptualization of place engagement as both a stressor and a protective factor in the prevention of illness. The Tribal Health Sovereignty model also calls for health researchers to center place and environment as health within Indigenous obesity prevention efforts (Jennings et al., 2018). In fact, culturally grounded, strengths-based interventions that center on local Indigenous knowledge, are effective at improving health and often, more accepted within communities (Fiedeldey-Van Dijk et al., 2017; Jennings et al., 2018; King, 2011; Rowan et al., 2014; Walters et al., 2018). Such interventions focus on positive tenets of both traditional and contemporary Indigenous cultures including connectedness through relationships with people and places (Fiedeldey-Van Dijk et al., 2017; Jennings et al., 2018; Mohatt et al., 2011).

This article focuses on relationship to place among NCIW who participated in *Yappalli: Choctaw Road to Health*, an experiential, land-based intervention that involved walking the physical path of the Choctaw Trail of Tears (Walters et al., 2018). The "Trail of Tears" is a major HTE that involved forced removal of five tribal nations under a federally mandated Indian removal policy in the 1830s. On the Choctaw Trail of Tears, over 12,500 Choctaw people were forced to walk 500 miles from their traditional homelands or face losing their tribal sovereignty (Barnett, 2012). An estimated amount of 2,500–6,000 people died from disease, starvation, and exposure (Akers, 2004; DeRosier, 1970; Foreman, 1932; Wright, 1928). This initial pilot study demonstrated how physically being in places where HTE occurred – even for NCIW as people from tribal communities other than the one in which the HTE occurred – was a multi-faceted process that illuminated experiences of both stress and resilience. While Choctaw women's physical experiences of re-walking the Trail of Tears have initially been analyzed and discussed (Schultz et al., 2016), the experiences of NCIW in the pilot study have remained unexamined. Physically walking the Choctaw Trail of Tears helped the NCIW connect with the trauma of their own tribal histories, and simultaneously develop transformative narratives of resilience.

Methods

Secondary qualitative data belonging to the four non-Choctaw Indigenous women were drawn from *Yappalli: Choctaw Road to Health*, a community-based, participatory pilot study (n = 12; Walters, Principal Investigator (PI) and Johnson-Jennings, Co-PI) conducted in 2012. In response to high rates of obesity and related adverse health outcomes among members of the Choctaw Nation of Oklahoma (CNO), Choctaw women researchers, community and academic, developed a pilot project incorporating culturally generative activities deeply rooted in relationship to place in order to develop an initial Choctaw health framework (see Walters et al., 2018). While Choctaw participants were recruited, non-Choctaw Indigenous volunteers were also recruited to provide support on the Trail and serve as witnesses. The non-Choctaw volunteers joined in re-walking the Choctaw Trail of Tears and participated in the curriculum regarding the place-based trauma and Choctaw ancestral teachings of hope and resilience.

Four Indigenous researchers, including the PI and co-PI Choctaw tribal members, took part in the trail experience as both participants and data collectors. They conducted semi-structured, in-depth, English-language interviews, and two focus groups among all Choctaw and Indigenous participants. All 12 Indigenous participants were recruited using convenience sampling, yielding a primarily female-identified sample for the pilot study. Utilizing a semi-structured interview guide that assessed new insights and reflections on health behaviors and attitudes within the context of experiences on the Trail, researchers collected data through in-depth interviews at pre-walk and post-walk, and focus groups conducted during the walk. This article analyzes the three months post-walk interviews from a total of four adult NCIW volunteers (one of whom was both an NCIW interviewer and participant). The post-walk interview guide included explicit questions related to experiences of place, which were the focus of this analysis. Additionally, any references to the place and health relationship within the entire transcripts were also analyzed. The specific place-related questions consisted of the following: 1) Were there any moments on the trail you felt connected to place? What was that like? Where did it happen? 2) If at all, how did the trail affect your sense of home? How did you feel that in your body? an example of open-ended health-related questions is "What does health and being healthy mean for you as a Native or Indigenous person, especially now that you have walked the trail?" The study received Institutional Review Board approval from both the University of Washington and the CNO to ensure the protection of human subjects. Schultz et al. (2016) and Walters et al. (2018) provide a more detailed description of the pilot study.

The NCIW in this sample were in their 20s and 30s, represented four distinct Indigenous nations of binational (U.S. and another country) origin, had graduate-level educations, and were working in health research. With phenomenology as our guiding methodology, we used an inductive, thematic analytic approach to capturing NCIW's embodied, lived experiences (Guest et al., 2012; Smith et al., 2009; Starks & Brown Trinidad, 2007). A sample size of four is within the typical range for phenomenological studies (Starks & Brown Trinidad, 2007), which aim to find a relatively homogenous sample in order to capture detailed, nuanced experiences (Smith et al., 2009). The metatheoretical assumptions of the ISCM (Walters et al., 2002) – the theoretical model that guides this study – are predicated upon Indigenous worldviews, which emphasize a relational worldview of interconnectedness, respect, and interdependence of both animate and inanimate things/beings. Additionally, the relational worldview recognizes one's role in maintaining balance and harmony in relationship with the natural environment and corresponding ancestral obligations (i.e., past and future generations) tied to the natural world, sacred sites, and original territories. Such relational worldviews are holistic and emphasize application to daily living in mutuality, respect, and mindfulness. Phenomenology guides the generation of themes and categories from NCIW narratives in order to illuminate individual and collective meanings of the NCIW experiences on the Trail, through embodied perception (Guest et al., 2012; Smith et al., 2009; Starks & Brown Trinidad, 2007).

This qualitative, thematic analytic approach included several steps that involved de-contextualization and re-contextualization within and across cases to narrow down the data to representative categories and organize it into clusters of representative meaning (Ayres et al., 2003). The lead author conducted all of the data analysis, with review and input by research study PIs, staff, and faculty. Initial coding began with data immersion through multiple readings of each transcript, followed by an analysis of individual transcripts and identification of keywords, phrases, sentences, and paragraphs that mention place, health, and the relationship between place and health. Next, intermediate coding involved a deeper analysis of the relationships between codes, leading to the generation of categories to create a codebook, which helped organize the data (Guest et al., 2012; Saldaña, 2009). Further coding occurred in Dedoose, a qualitative analytics software, in order to generate a coherent, engaging story that illuminates deep understanding of participant experiences with health and place as contextually grounded (Ayres et al., 2003).

To ensure rigor and trustworthiness, the lead author acknowledged their insider/outsider status as an NCIW who participated as a volunteer in a sequential NIH funded randomized control trial for a Yappalli health intervention, several years after the pilot study analyzed in this article was conducted. The lead author also worked with some participants and members of the research team on different projects before and after the pilot study. Thus, even with de-identified data, there were instances where the lead author recognized participants based on their narratives. However, those relationships with participants and members of the research team enabled the lead author to triangulate the data and engage in member checking. The lead author engaged in memo-writing and consultation with the research staff and faculty in order to bracket personal biases and perspectives (Corbin Dwyer & Buckle, 2009). Furthermore, all of the coauthors except for the second author participated in the Yappalli pilot study.

Results

Two main themes emerged from the analysis, each with two sub-themes. First, the NCIW experienced *stress embodied* which reflected the visceral connection to the Choctaw Trail of Tears as well as subthemes of feeling connected to ancestral trauma and the recognition of its impact on contemporary health disparities. Second, *resilience embodied* reflected the NCIW reconstructed narratives of the transformation of trauma to health, through subthemes of connectedness to place, and through forging a collective path of resistance for future generations.

Stress embodied: "Being on the walk put it somewhere in my body"

Drawing on concepts of historical trauma and its manifestation in contemporary health adversities, NCIW connected specific HTEs that resulted in or from environmental dispossession – including forced relocations, compulsory attendance of boarding schools, and loss of traditional knowledge – to contemporary health disparities, disconnection from identity and land, and violence. NCIW narratives revealed the physical and emotional stress they experienced as they reflected on the intergenerational impacts of such HTEs. One NCIW related her own family's premature deaths from chronic disease, with an understanding now on a corporeal level:

> Every single year, at least one of my relatives has died of these things, so going through that as a relative has been hard and arduous and painful. Being on the walk put it somewhere in my body, an understanding that is now in my cells.

Another NCIW described her visceral reaction as she recognized the connection between historical trauma and contemporary health outcomes on the Trail:

> A lot of the traumas that were experienced 100 … 200 years ago, are still happening … It makes me feel sick. It takes away energy. It feels really heavy … it's historically situated, but it extends into the present moment, like a spider web … the reasons that our people are getting sick and dying, they're the same reasons as they were.

Historical trauma: "It's historically situated"

Although NCIW recognized differences in HTE across the Choctaw and their own tribal nations, they also saw numerous connections. NCIW shared their own experiences of pain and grief surrounding the trauma of the Choctaw Trail of Tears. One NCIW described how walking with Choctaw participants on the Trail deepened her own connection to historical trauma: "There's sort of this peripheral awareness of the atrocities that were committed against Choctaws and against native communities .... to really have to face it in a tangible way made me really have to connect to that trauma differently."

The clear physical impact of thousands of Indigenous footsteps on the Choctaw Trail of Tears was striking and evoked visceral reactions in NCIW. One portion of the Trail in what is now known as Village Creek State Park, Arkansas, was sunken six to ten feet below ground level by the thousands of Indigenous people forced to walk the Trail of Tears. One NCIW recounted her reaction to this site: "I really feel pain in my heart .... I feel shock .... We hurt ... I hurt."

This NCIW's description is an example of how the impact of trauma from a place is more than symbolic – the sunken path was a powerful, physical reminder of the thousands of men, women, and children whose footsteps literally shaped the Choctaw Trail of Tears. She recollected her own tribal history of politically imposed violence, and highlighted the connectedness of Indigenous experiences across the globe:

> Even though it is not in my history, this happened in different ways in different parts of the world. We also experienced violence policies like relocation. I feel like we are very similar so I would like to join. ... I believe that other Indigenous people, if they visit [her tribal nation], they may have this kind of feeling.

Contemporary trauma: "It extends into the present moment"

NCIW described how historical trauma manifests in contemporary traumas, via embodied health disparities rooted in environmental dispossession. One NCIW explained how confinement to reservations and compulsory boarding school attendance played a role in the dispossession from traditional foods:

> A lot of folks who ended up with commodity foods or who were taken away no longer had the ability to gather traditional foods and hunt. It clearly has to do with the levels of poor health, obesity, and diabetes that we see in our communities now.

Finding ways to release emotional pain resulting from such environmental dispossession is a natural response to trauma, and may be evident in behaviors leading to either disease or health. One NCIW described alcohol as one pathway for pain release in her tribal community: "... historical trauma affects contemporary disease. During the walk, a lot of us carry the pain, and we need somewhere to release the pain …. drinking alcohol in my community is the way people try to release the pain." Another NCIW not only recognized the impact of trauma embodied on personal and communal illness but also her ability to heal: "Holding things in your body will make you sick. It definitely used to make me sick, and I've learned ways to not hold it into my body as much."

Resilience embodied: "Because of them, we're still here"

These NCIW's stories describe not only how trauma is transmitted across generations, from cell to society, but also the intergenerational pathways of resilience. Through embodying their own Indigenous definitions of health as individual, communal, and place connectedness, and through resisting ongoing colonially imposed adversities, NCIW narratives demonstrated resilience embodied. Inspired by the Choctaw participants' ancestral visions of health and resilience, walking on the Choctaw Trail of Tears helped NCIW connect with their own tribal ancestors' strength and resilience. One NCIW recognized this intergenerational transmission of resilience:

> … we're here because of them and what they gave up for us. They had to deal with all of the hardships and straight-on trauma … .They were resilient and able to stay here. Because of them, we're still here even though there's not as many of us anymore …

Connectedness to place is health: "Health means … the place that you're in"

NCIW narratives frame health as a multidimensional sense of connectedness across tribes, generations, and places – whether those places are their own or others' ancestral lands. One NCIW explained: "health means more than just what is happening to your body … your experiences, your ancestors' experiences, the place that you're in, the people you're interacting with, the way you're interacting with them, all of those things influence health." Another NCIW summarized the connection with the natural environment as part of the Indigenous community – a connection that facilitates multi-dimensional, multi-generational relationships:

> When I have a chance to connect with people, I will have a chance to connect with the environment … And if I connect it with the environment, it will be easy for me to connect with the other generations, with the ancestors, with what happened there.

This multidimensional, expansive conceptualization of health as connectedness is prominent across all of the interviews. These connections can be made, maintained, and strengthened through cultural and spiritual practices that reinforce Indigenous identity and provide a coping mechanism to heal from trauma. Another NCIW described how she releases her trauma through practices which themselves can create places of prevention – practices grounded in teachings about the natural environment: "I have [cultural dance form], we have ceremonies, we have medicines, so I don't have to carry it with me all the time."

A shared path of resistance: "We're trying to create ... a path that was healing"

Resisting in place – whether through re-walking the Choctaw Trail of Tears or through participating in cultural and spiritual practices that create and reinforce place connections – was viewed as key to multigenerational pre-servation of Indigenous health. One NCIW explains: "We're still recovering from colonial processes, and this walk is part of that decolonizing work." She describes how walking the Choctaw Trail of Tears transformed it from a path of trauma and health disparities to a "shared path of resistance:"

> This is, this will be my life's work ... to shift this, to transform this ... . the new Trail of Tears as the health disparities we're all dying from ... . Just the fact that we were there doing this, that you were all doing this especially meant that it was changing.

Cultural and spiritual practices that create and reinforce a connection to place were considered an "antidote" to contemporary traumas, which one NCIW defined as "trying to be healthy and well, having movement, [dance], eating well, going to ceremonies, and trying to learn our Indigenous lan-guages." Reclaiming these practices involved the adaptation and evolution of cultural practices, which is key to Indigenous resilience through the genera-tions. She further explained:

> There is a fierce resolution to be who we are regardless of where we get pushed to be ... our cultural traditions; our cultural symbols have changed over time and history, the essence is still the same ... this way that we maintain ourselves, our spirits, despite, colonial processes is what keeps us alive. We're fighting for our health and wellness.

One NCIW summarized the transformation that both NCIW and Choctaw participants experienced by walking on the Choctaw Trail of Tears, as a vision for the health of future generations: "We were trying to create more of a path that was healing versus remembering it as a path of trauma and trying to make it different for the next generations and the younger people."

Discussion

This is the first known study to examine how supporting a tribally specific HTE place-based healing journey influences the health views of Indigenous people from other tribal groupings. The key findings of this study include several themes that illuminate the power of being in places where HTE occurred. For NCIW, walking the Choctaw Trail of Tears evoked a visceral connection to both intergenerational stress and resilience (Dodge, 2007) that merely hearing or reading about the Choctaw Trail of Tears could not. NCIW drew connections between intergenerational, intertribal health disparities, and their origins in HTE that disrupted the place relationship. Walking the Trail of Tears in support of the Choctaw women evoked a sense of empathy and solidarity among NCIW, as they recognized the common threads of historical and contemporary trauma between the Choctaw and their own tribal histories. Simultaneously, walking the Trail of Tears connected them with a sense of intergenerational, intertribal resilience. Their reconstructed narratives demonstrated that place connection is integral to connections with ancestors, community, and future generations (Walters, Beltrán et al., 2011; Mohatt et al., 2011), ultimately shaping conceptualizations of health. As HTEs are linked to health inequities, strategies of resistance are linked to Indigenous wellness and healing. Walking the Choctaw Trail of Tears, for these NCIW, encompassed micro and communal acts of resistance (Evans-Campbell & Campbell, 2019). From their personal commitments to health and wellness, to their communal organization as a group of intertribal Indigenous women, re-tracing their Indigenous ancestors' footsteps, metaphorically, was their "life's work." While remaining in and retracing sites of destructive HTE can have adverse impacts on health and well-being (O'Neil, 1986), connecting with these same places can also facilitate narratives of "survivance" (Vizenor, 2008). These sites can be sources of healing and resilience where micro, communal, and political acts of resistance (Evans-Campbell & Campbell, 2019) are merged to transform trauma to healing. Furthermore, Indigenous women have a unique relationship to land: they embody resistance to settler colonialism as an ongoing, gendered process (Arvin et al., 2013). Moreover, in many tribal matrilineal societies, Indigenous women are responsible for or actively participate in restoring tribal well-being when a great trauma has occurred in addition to protecting and maintaining ongoing land-based ceremonial and agricultural practices and responsibilities (Pesantubbee, 2005).

Findings should be considered in light of the study's strengths and limitations. The strengths of this study include its innovative contribution to a neglected body of place-based Indigenous health literature. In addition, this study is a unique examination of the experiences of Indigenous peoples who voluntarily accompany descendants of survivors of a particular tribal nation and their tribally specific HTE to the physical site of the original trauma. Furthermore, the sample is comprised of NCIW who belong to four different Indigenous groups of binational origins (the U.S. and another country), at two different developmental stages in their 20 s and 30 s. Their distinct cultural perspectives cut across tribal specificity, a critical aspect for identifying common components that could be built into other Indigenous outdoor experiential health strategies. Yet, limitations may emerge from similar sample characteristics including gender, younger adult age grouping, educational level, and similar perspectives on health promotion and the role of historical trauma in health disparities. It is uncertain whether similar findings would emerge from a sample comprised broader gender, age, and career groups. Furthermore, one NCIW is both an interviewer/partici-pant – an insider/outsider positioned in a unique space of insight yet potential influence which must be bracketed as discussed in the Methods section (Corbin Dwyer & Buckle, 2009). These qualitative findings aim to identify more nuanced and often neglected issues rather than be representa-tive of the population. Future work could examine a larger sample in order to expand the range of in-depth perspectives that would help strengthen study saturation.

This study has important implications for theoretical expansion, interven-tion, and knowledge development necessary for culturally congruent social work practice with Indigenous people. Theoretical expansion might incorpo-rate additional dimensions to conceptual models such as the ISCM (Walters et al., 2002) in terms of the person–place relationship as both a source of stress (e.g., environmental dispossession) and resilience (e.g., participation in place-based cultural/spiritual activities). This expansion could be useful for developing and testing measures related to health and place using qualitative, quantitative, and mixed methods designs. Findings may also assist in the development of new models to inform interventions aimed at decreasing Indigenous peoples' health disparities. Additionally, conducting a future comparative analysis could shed light on differences and similarities between the experiences of Choctaw and NCIW participants on the Choctaw Trail of Tears. This may ultimately lead to a better understanding of experiences of intertribal participants in tribally specific HTE-related healing projects. Moreover, future research on the role of gender in understanding Indigenous health and place-based interventions is warranted. This study also has specific implications for the field of social work. It contributes to the paucity of literature on the role of place in Indigenous health, which brings ample opportunity for developing culturally relevant, settings-based holistic practice techniques and interventions. Furthermore, expanding the literature on the impact of social *and* environmental determinants of health should include the role of place relationships in health equity, especially in light of the increasing threats of climate change that disproportionately impact

Indigenous people globally (Billiot et al., 2019; Willox et al., 2013). Such efforts not only have significant implications for building crucial research infrastructure but also for addressing ecological health inequities through culturally and methodologically innovative approaches. Through looking at the various aspects of the place and health relationship for Indigenous people, we can reach a more nuanced understanding of both the etiological origins and pragmatic implications for the place and health relationship as we aim to combat health disparities and inequities among Indigenous peoples (Billiot et al., 2019). Walking on the Choctaw Trail of Tears provided a pathway of transformation for NCIW, shaping narratives of healing for themselves and future generations.

Acknowledgments

With gratitude to Dr. Jordan Lewis and Dr. Susan Kemp for their editorial assistance.

Disclosure statement

The authors reported no potential conflict of interest.

Funding

This work was supported, in part by the National Institutes of Health (NIH) National Institute on Drug Abuse Grant 1R01DA037176 and Contract HHSN271201200663P, and the National Institute on Minority Health and Health Disparities Grant P60MD006909. This work was also supported in part by the Substance Abuse and Mental Health Services Administration Grant 5T06SM060560.

ORCID

Angela R. Fernandez ⓘ http://orcid.org/0000-0001-9066-7367

References

Akers, D. (2004). *Living in the land of death: The Choctaw nation*. Michigan State University Press.

Alfred, T., & Corntassel, J. (2005). Being indigenous: Resurgences against contemporary colonialism. *Government and Opposition*, *40*(4), 597–614. https://doi.org/10.1111/j.1477-7053.2005.00166.x

Arvin, M., Tuck, E., & Morrill, A. (2013). Decolonizing feminism: Challenging connections between settler colonialism and heteropatriarchy. *Feminist Formations*, *25*(1), 8–34. https://doi.org/10.1353/ff.2013.0006

Ayres, L., Kavanaugh, K., & Knafl, K. A. (2003). Within-case and across-case approaches to qualitative data analysis. *Qualitative Health Research*, *13*(6), 871–883. https://doi.org/10.1177/1049732303013006008

Barnett, J. F., Jr. (2012). *Mississippi's American Indians*. University Press of Mississippi.

Beltrán, R., Schultz, K., Fernández, A., Walters, K., Duran, B., & Evans-Campbell, T. (2018). From ambivalence to revitalization: Negotiating cardiovascular health behaviors related to environmental and historical trauma in a Northwest American Indian community. *American Indian and Alaska Native Mental Health Research*, 25(2), 103–128. https://doi.org/10.5820/aian.2502.2018.103

Billiot, S., Beltrán, R., Mitchell, F., Brown, D., & Fernández, A. (2019). Indigenous perspectives for strengthening social responses to global environmental changes: A response to the social work grand challenge on environmental change. *Journal of Community Practice*, 27(3–4), 296–316. https://doi.org/10.1080/10705422.2019.1658677

Brave Heart, M. Y. H., Chase, J., Elkins, J., & Altschul, D. B. (2011). Historical trauma among Indigenous peoples of the Americas: Concepts, research, and clinical considerations. *Journal of Psychoactive Drugs*, 43(4), 282–290. https://doi.org/10.1080/02791072.2011.628913

Calloway, C. G. (2008). *First peoples: A documentary survey of American Indian history* (3rd ed.). Bedford/St. Martin's.

Corbin Dwyer, S., & Buckle, J. L. (2009). The space between: On being an insider-outsider in qualitative research. *International Journal of Qualitative Methods*, 8(1), 54–63. https://doi.org/10.1177/160940690900800105

DeRosier, A. H. (1970). *The removal of the Choctaw Indians*. University of Tennessee Press.

Dodge, W. A. (2007). Introduction to place-making, identity, and cultural landscapes. In W. A. Dodge (Ed.), *Black rock: A Zuni cultural landscape and the meaning of place* (pp. 3–16). University Press of Mississippi.

Evans-Campbell, T., & Campbell, C. (2019). Indigenist oppression and resistance in Indian child welfare: Reclaiming our children. In J. H. Schiele (Ed.), *Social welfare policy: Regulation and resistance among people of color* (2nd ed., pp. 295–313). Cognella Press.

Evans-Campbell, T., & Walters, K. L. (2006). Catching our breath: A decolonization framework for healing indigenous families. In R. Fong, R. McRoy, & C. Ortiz Hendricks (Eds.), *Intersecting child welfare, substance abuse, and family violence: Culturally competent approaches* (pp. 266–292). CSWE Publications.

Fernandez, A. R. (2019). Wherever I go, I have it inside of me: Indigenous cultural dance as a transformative place of health and prevention for members of an urban Danza Mexica community (Publication No. 22620258) [Doctoral dissertation, University of Washington]. Proquest Dissertations and Theses Global.

Fiedeldey-Van Dijk, C., Rowan, M., Dell, C., Mushquash, C., Hopkins, C., Fornssler, B., Hall, L., Mykota, D., Farag, M., & Shea, B. (2017). Honoring indigenous culture-as-intervention: Development and validity of the native wellness assessment. *Journal of Ethnicity in Substance Abuse*, 16(2), 181–218. https://doi.org/10.1080/15332640.2015.1119774

First Nations Development Institute. (2013). *Reclaiming native food systems: Part I*.

Foreman, G. (1932). *Indian removal: The emigration of the five civilized tribes of Indians*. University of Oklahoma Press.

Guest, G., MacQueen, K. M., & Namey, E. E. (2012). *Applied thematic analysis*. Sage Publications.

Hoover, E., Cook, K., Plain, R., Sanchez, V., Waghiyi, V., Miller, P., Dufault, R., Sislin, C., & Carpenter, D. O. (2012). Indigenous peoples of North America: Environmental exposures and reproductive justice. *Environmental Health Perspectives*, 120(12), 1645–1649. https://doi.org/10.1289/ehp.1205422

Jennings, D. M., Little, M., & Johnson-Jennings, M. (2018). Developing a tribal health sovereignty model for obesity prevention as guided by photovoice. *Progress in

Community Health Partnerships Research Education and Action, 12(3), 353–362. https://doi.org/10.1353/cpr.2018.0059

King, J. (2011). Reclaiming our roots: Accomplishments and challenges. *Journal of Psychoactive Drugs, 43*(3), 297–301. https://doi.org/10.1080/02791072.2011.628921

Kirmayer, L. J., Dandeneau, S., Marshall, E., Phillips, M. K., & Williamson, K. J. (2011). Rethinking resilience from Indigenous perspectives. *Canadian Journal of Psychiatry, 56*(2), 84–91. https://doi.org/10.1177/070674371105600203

Krieger, N. (2005). Embodiment: A conceptual glossary for epidemiology. *Journal of Epidemiology and Community Health (1979-), 59*(5), 350–355. https://doi.org/10.1136/jech.2004.024562

Krieger, N., & Davey Smith, G. (2004). "Bodies count," and body counts: Social epidemiology and embodying inequality. *Epidemiologic Reviews, 26*(1), 92–103. https://doi.org/10.1093/epirev/mxh009

Lewis, J., Hoover, J., & MacKenzie, D. (2017). Mining and environmental health disparities in Native American communities. *Current Environmental Health Reports, 4*(2), 130–141. https://doi.org/10.1007/s40572-017-0140-5

Mohatt, N. V., Fok, C. C. T., Burket, R., Henry, D., & Allen, J. (2011). Assessment of awareness of connectedness as a culturally-based protective factor for Alaska Native youth. *Cultural Diversity & Ethnic Minority Psychology, 17*(4), 444–455. https://doi.org/10.1037/a0025456

O'Neil, J. D. (1986). The politics of health in the Fourth World: A northern Canadian example. *Human Organization, 45*(2), 119–128. https://doi.org/10.17730/humo.45.2.q34m761r857km8lh

Pesantubbee, M. (2005). *Choctaw women in a chaotic world: The clash of cultures in the colonial Southeast.* University of New Mexico Press.

Ramirez, R. K. (2007). *Native hubs: Culture, community, and belonging in Silicon Valley and beyond.* Duke University Press.

Richmond, C. A. M., & Ross, N. A. (2009). The determinants of First Nation and inuit health: A critical population health approach. *Health & Place, 15*(2), 403–411. https://doi.org/10.1016/j.healthplace.2008.07.004

Rowan, M., Poole, N., Shea, B., Gone, J. P., Mykota, D., Farag, Farag, M., Hopkins, C., Hall, L., Mushquash, C., & Dell, C. (2014). Cultural interventions to treat addictions in Indigenous populations: Findings from a scoping study. *Substance Abuse Treatment, Prevention, and Policy, 9*(1), 34–59. https://doi.org/10.1186/1747-597X-9-34

Saldaña, J. (2009). *The coding manual for qualitative researchers.* Sage Publications.

Schultz, K., Walters, K. L., Beltrán, R., Stroud, S., & Johnson-Jennings, M. (2016). "I'm stronger than I thought": Native women reconnecting to body, health, and place. *Health and Place, 40*, 21–28. https://doi.org/http://doi.10.1016/j.healthplace.2016.05.001

Smith, J. A., Flowers, P., & Larkin, M. (2009). *Interpretive phenomenological analysis: Theory, method and research.* Sage Publications Ltd.

Sotero, M. M. (2006). A conceptual model of historical trauma: Implications for public health practice and research. *Journal of Health Disparities Research and Practice, 1*, 93–108. https://ssrn.com/abstract=1350062

Starks, H., & Brown Trinidad, S. (2007). Choose your method: A comparison of phenomenology, discourse analysis, and grounded theory. *Qualitative Health Research, 17*(10), 1372–1380. https://doi.org/10.1177/1049732307307031

Vizenor, G. R. (2008). *Survivance: Narratives of native presence.* University of Nebraska Press.

Vukic, A., Gregory, D., Martin-Misener, R., & Etowa, J. (2011). Aboriginal and western conceptions of mental health and illness. *Pimatisiwin: A Journal of Aboriginal &*

Indigenous Community Health, 9(1), 65–86. http://www.pimatisiwin.com/online/wp-con tent/uploads/2011/08/04VukicGregory.pdf

Walters, K. L., Beltrán, R. E., Huh, D., & Evans-Campbell, T. (2011). Dis-placement and disease: Land, place and health among American Indians and Alaska natives. In L. M. Burton, S. P. Kemp, M. Leung, S. A. Matthews, & D. T. Takeuchi (Eds.), *Communities, neighborhood, and health: Expanding the boundaries of place* (pp. 163–199). Springer Science +Business Media, LLC.

Walters, K. L., Johnson-Jennings, M. K., Stroud, S. A., Rasmus, S. W., Charles, B. O., John, S., & Boulafentis, J. (2018). Growing from our roots: Strategies for developing culturally grounded health promotion interventions in American Indian, Alaska native, and Native Hawaiian communities. *Prevention Science,* 21(Suppl 1): 1–11. https://doi.org/10.1007/ s11121-018-0952-z

Walters, K. L., Mohammed, S. A., Evans-Campbell, T., Beltrán, R. E., Chae, D. H., & Duran, B. (2011). Bodies don't just tell stories, they tell histories: Embodiment of historical trauma among American Indians and Alaska natives. *Du Bois Review, 8*(1), 179–189. https://doi.org/10.1017/S1742058X1100018X

Walters, K. L., & Simoni, J. M. (2002). Reconceptualizing native women's health: An "indigenist" stress-coping model. *American Journal of Public Health, 92*(4), 520–524. https://doi.org/10.2105/AJPH.92.4.520

Walters, K. L., Simoni, J. M., & Evans-Campbell, T. (2002). Substance use among American Indians and Alaska natives: Incorporating culture in an "Indigenist" stress-coping paradigm. *Public Health Reports,* 117(1), 104–117. https://pubmed.ncbi.nlm.nih.gov/12435834/

Whitbeck, L. B., Adams, G. W., Hoyt, D. R., & Chen, X. (2004). Conceptualizing and measuring historical trauma among American Indian people. *American Journal of Community Psychology, 33*(3–4), 119–130. https://doi.org/10.1023/B:AJCP.0000027000. 77357.31

Willox, C., Harper, E., Landman, H., & Ford, & the Rigolet Inuit Community Government. (2013). The land enriches the soul: On climatic and environmental change, affect and emotional health and well-being in Rigolet, Nunatsiavut, Canada. *Emotion, Space and Society, 6*(2013), 14–24. https://doi.org/10.1016/j.emospa.2011.08.005

Wright, M. H. (1928). The removal of the Choctaws to the Indian territory, 1830–1833. *Chronicles of Oklahoma, 6*(2), 103–128. https://scholar.google.com/scholar_lookup?jour nal=Chronicles+of+Oklahoma&title=The+removal+of+the+Choctaws+to+the+Indian +Territory,+1830%E2%80%931833&author=MH+Wright&volume=6&issue=2&publica tion_year=1928&pages=103-128&

The development and testing of a multi-level, multi-component pilot intervention to reduce sexual and reproductive health disparities in a tribal community

Elizabeth Rink, Mike Anastario, Olivia Johnson, Ramey GrowingThunder, Paula Firemoon, Adriann Ricker, Genevieve Cox, and Shannon Holder

ABSTRACT

This manuscript presents the results from a multi- level, multi-component pilot intervention designed to reduce sexual and reproductive health (SRH) among American Indian (AI) youth living on a reservation in the Northwestern United States. Our theoretical framework included community based participatory research (CBPR) and Ecological Systems Theory (EST). The pilot intervention was a school-based curriculum for youth and parents and a cultural mentoring program. Mixed methods were used including a pre/post test design and focus groups. Quantitative data was analyzed using McNemar's chi-square and a random effects model. Qualitative data was analyzed with grounded theory and content analysis. Parents reported increased communication about SRH topics with their children. Youth reported increased condom use self-efficacy, increased condom use, and positive agreement with attitudes toward pregnancy. Our results also suggest increased communication about SRH topics in parent dyads and the need for increased communication with elders. Future research is needed to test the efficacy of multi-level, multi-component tribally driven SRH interventions for AI youth and their families that integrate contemporary SRH issues with traditional values and beliefs.

Introduction

American Indian (AI) populations have disproportionately high sexual and reproductive health (SRH) disparities (Centers for Disease Control and Prevention [CDC], 2014). Teen births, pre-term birth, low birth weight, miscarriages and ectopic pregnancies, and sexually transmitted infections (STIs) are much higher in AIs compared to other racial and ethnic populations (CDC, 2013, 2014). Also, the incidence of HIV and HCV in AI populations in the United States continues to rise (CDC, 2017a).

Current literature suggests that the experiences of Colonialization that AI populations have endured in the United States, such as sexual violence and rape, theft of land use and water rights, family denigration through boarding schools, the criminalization of cultural practices and forced sterilization of AI women, inform their SRH disparities (Arnold, 2014; Gurr, 2012). In addition, poverty, isolation, alcohol and other drug use, physical and sexual victimization, and lack of comprehensive and coordinated SRH education and clinical services influence unintended pregnancies and STIs in AI communities (De Ravello et al., 2014; Whitesell et al., 2014). Evidence also suggests that ambivalence toward sex, social pressures, depression, and anxiety among AIs contribute to their poor SRH outcomes (Hanson et al., 2014).

This collective body of knowledge highlights that SRH among AI population is influenced by the combination of individual, historical, structural, and community dynamics. Thus, to improve SRH outcomes in AI populations, novel multi-level interventions are needed (Tingey et al., 2017). This manuscript presents the results from a multi- level, multi-component pilot intervention designed to reduce SRH among AI youth ages 15 to 18 years old. The purpose of this study was to refine and tailor a pilot intervention for a larger clinical trial with AI youth and their families on a reservation.

Pilot intervention model

Community based participatory research

Our pilot intervention was built on a 14-year partnership using community based participatory research (CBPR) between a tribal community in the Northern Plains and outside non-Indigenous researchers from a land grant research institution (Rink et al., 2016). Central to our use of CBPR was a community advisory board (CAB) and a tribal and outside non-Indigenous research team that worked collaboratively to design and implement the pilot intervention. The CAB provided oversight and guidance for the pilot intervention and included five tribal members representing an equitable distribution of gender, age and tribal affiliation reflective of the community in which the pilot intervention was conducted. The tribal research team consisted of three full to part time paid staff. There were two outside non-Indigenous researchers.

Pilot intervention design

Our pilot intervention was developed in collaboration with the CAB and the tribal and outside non-Indigenous research team. Over 12 months meetings were held to review and discuss our current data on the tribal youth that was gathered during an exploratory study that took place to identify community needs. Existing literature on SRH interventions was also reviewed and discussed by the CAB and research team. Based on this iterative, collaborative process the three levels of the pilot intervention were designed using Ecological Systems Theory (Table 1) (Bronfenbrenner, 1999).

The individual level component included the implementation of the school based SRH curriculum for AI youth called *Native Stand*. For the purpose of our pilot intervention, *Native Stand* was adapted from a 28-module SRH curriculum to 18-module. Content focused on SRH topics that were relevant to a tribal and culturally context in addition to general SRH education. Examples of topics addressed in *Native Stand* were culture and tradition, healthy relationships, and pregnancy and parenting within a tribal context, negotiation and refusal skills and effective communication. The family level component was based on an adaptation of *Native Voices* that was originally designed for AI youth. For the purposes of our pilot intervention we adapted 5 modules from *Native Voices* into 3 modules. The 3 *Native Voices* modules provided education to parents regarding how to communicate with their children about sensitive topics such as sex, condom and birth control use, and STIs. The community level component involved a cultural mentoring program that was designed by the tribal language and culture program. The cultural mentoring program provided male and female elders to mentor youth participating in the pilot intervention in traditional values, beliefs and practices related to kinship networks and concepts of family and genealogy, male/female roles and beliefs about healthy relationships, and cultural beliefs about sex and how to make decisions about sex that integrate traditional values.

The pilot intervention took place over 9 weeks. During the 9-week period *Native Stand* was implemented twice a week. *Native Voices* was implemented three times at the tribal community school in the early evening. The cultural mentoring program was implemented in small groups during the class periods that *Native Stand* was taught. As incentives, the youth received 10.00 USD Google Play or I-Tunes cards and the parents received 20.00 USD gift cards to a local convenience store.

Table 1. Pilot intervention conceptual model.

Community Based Participatory Research Process				
Community Identifies Needs *10 focus groups * 29 key informants * Discussions with tribal leadership	**Develop Ecological Systems Theory Framework** * A holistic approach to SRH: indvidual, family, community	**Design and Implement Pilot Intervention** * Pre/post test with youth and parents	**Evaluate Pilot Intervention** * 2 focus groups with youth and parents * Analysis of pilot data	**Determine Next Steps for Behavioral Health Interventi**
Ecological Systems Theory Framework of Intervention				
Individual Level **Native Stand**		**Family Level** **Native Voices**	**Community Level** **Cultural Mentoring Program**	
18 session school based curriculum twice a week (NS)		*3 sessions delivered to parents in the early evening (NV)*	*3 cultural mentoring sessions delivered in small groups during class periods (CM)*	
NS 1: Introduction NS 2: Culture & Tradition – Part 1 NS 3: Culture & Tradition – Part 2 NS 4: Healthy Relationships – Part 1 NS 5: Healthy Relationships – Part 2		NV 1: Introduction and talking with youth about topics related to sexual and reproductive health	CMP 1: Kinship networks and concepts of family and genealogy	
NS 6: Reproductive Health – Part 1 NS 7: Reproductive Health – Part 2 NS 8: Pregnancy & Parenting NS 9: Preventing Pregnancy NS 10: Condoms and Birth Control NS 11: Sexually Transmitted Diseases		NV 2: Strategies for fostering healthy relationships in your child's intimate relationships	CMP 2: Traditional male/female roles and Cultural beliefs about healthy relationships	
NS 12: HIV/AIDS & HCV NS 13: Drugs & Alcohol & Sex NS 14: Mental Health & Sex NS 15: Negotiation & Refusal Skills NS 16: Decision Making NS 17: Effective Communication NS 18: Putting It All Together		NV 3: Prevention of STIs, HIV/AIDs and HCV	CMP 3: Cultural beliefs about sex and how to make decisions about sex that integrate cultural values	

Materials and methods

Data collection

The pilot intervention took place on a reservation in the north western United States in one of the reservation's smaller communities (population 225). The CAB suggested this particular setting because they believed the community's small size would be instrumental in assisting with understanding the processes necessary to take when implementing a complex intervention. Youth and parents participating in the pilot intervention completed pre- and posttest surveys. Feedback on the pilot intervention was provided in two separate focus groups.

Sample and recruitment

In total, 17 youth participated in *Native Stand* and 12 parents participated in *Native Voices*. The youth and parents all completed pre-and post-intervention surveys. Two homogenously composed focus groups were conducted at the end of intervention's implementation to get feedback on the strengths and weaknesses of the intervention content. One focus group included 6 youth who participated in the intervention and completed the student pre-post intervention survey. The other focus group included 4 parents who participated in the intervention and completed the parent pre-post intervention survey. The youth and parent participants all identified as AI. This sample size represented half of the total population of youth and their parents between the ages of 15 – 18 attending school in this community.

The youth and parents were drawn from the high school located in the community where the intervention was taking place using purposive selection. The members of the tribal research team worked closely with school administration and teachers to present and discuss the study and identify the most appropriate ways to approach youth and their parents to participate in the pilot intervention. The members of the tribal research team approached the youth in the 10th, 11th, and 12th grades during their health class to talk about the pilot intervention and answer questions. Parents were mailed letters to their homes with information about the pilot intervention. In addition a parent meeting during after school hours was held to inform parents about the pilot intervention and to provide the parents an opportunity to ask questions to the tribal research team. Written consent was received from both the youth and their parent for youth participation in the study. Parents gave written consent for their participation. Youth and their parents were told they could withdraw from the study at any time. Institutional Review Board (IRB) approval for the study obtained from outside-non-Indigenous researchers home institution and the tribal IRB. The tribal IRB also reviewed and approved this manuscript for publication.

Questionnaires

The parent and youth questionnaires were administered prior to and immediately following the completion of the pilot intervention. Parent questionnaires included items on SRH topics they communicated about with their child/children. Youth questionnaire included items measuring sexual risk behaviors, parent/legal guardian communication, cultural identity, self-efficacy regarding condom use and birth control, knowledge and attitudes regarding pregnancy, healthcare accessibility, mental health and substance use. Our primary outcome measure was the ratio of condom use frequency relative to sexual intercourse frequency in the 30 days preceding questionnaire administration (Tingey et al., 2017). Questionnaires were administered using Computer Assisted Self Interview (CASI) (Ghanem et al., 2005).

Measures

The measures used in this study are presented in Table 2. Due to the limited sample size, individual items are reported for each measurement domain instead of reducing the number of items using factor analysis or other item-reduction techniques.

Focus groups

Following the completion of the pilot intervention, two focus groups were conducted by a member of the CAB. Open-ended questions were asked about the strengths and the challenges of the pilot

Table 2. Summary of data collection measures for student and parent survey.

Measure	Reference	Number of Items	Description
Youth Survey			
Attitudes regarding hypothetical pregnancy	(Mitchell et al., 2000)	13 items	Three-point Likert Scale *1 = Disagree, 3 = Agree*
Self-efficacy regarding condom use	(Beckman et al., 1992)	12 items	Five-point Likert Scale *1 = Not at all confident, 5 = Extremely confident*
Sexual risk behavior: Ratio of condom use to sexual engagement	(Bernstein et al., 2012)	2 items	Number of times of sex in past month Number of times condom was used in past month
Depression symptoms over past week	(Haroz et al., 2014)	10 items	*0 = 0 days, 1 = 1–2 days 2 = 3–4 days 3 = 5–7 days*
Substance use	(CDC, 2017b)	8 items	Sum of one-month history using alcohol, marijuana, meth, cocaine, ecstasy, heroin, steroids, and inhalants
Demographic information		4 items	Gender, age, town, sexuality
Parent Survey			
Parent/legal guardian-child SRH communication	(Beckett et al., 2010)	25 items	*1 = Yes, 0 = No*
Global ability to communicate with child and ability to communicate about sex	(Jerman & Constantine, 2010)	3 items	Five-point Likert Scale *1 = Difficult, 5 = Easy*
Demographic information		4 items	Gender, age, highest education completed, marital status

intervention, perceived changes in youth behavior, the cultural mentoring component of the intervention, and experiences completing the pre- and posttest questionnaires. All focus group participants consented to participation. The focus groups were recorded and transcribed.

Data analysis

Quantitative and qualitative data were used in our pilot intervention. Quantitative data were analyzed using STATA 14 statistical software (StataCorp, 2015). Parent and youth datasets were separately examined to determine scores on key domains prior to (pre) and following (post) implementation of the intervention. McNemar's chi-square test was used to evaluate relationships between dichotomous communication measures pre- and post-intervention. Each variable with a Likert scale response set was evaluated using a random effects model, where random effects were specified for the constant (individual youth or parents). Due to the small sample size and the pilot nature of this project, we examined the relative direction of beta values and standard errors of the estimates and focused less on a statistical significance criterion.

For the qualitative research, we used grounded theory to systematically code and analyze data for emergent themes (Corbin & Strauss, 2008). The focus group transcripts were coded in Atlas.ti (ATLAS. ti). One coder used open codes to develop a set of axial codes. These axial codes were shared and discussed between the CAB, the tribal and the non-Indigenous research team. Changes in the axial codes based on this discussion were given back to the coder to develop new axial codes. Themes were then developed that were again discussed with the CAB, the tribal and the non-Indigenous research team. Based on this discussion, the coder finalized the themes that that were then used to write the qualitative results section of the manuscript. This iterative, inclusive process ensured that themes in the qualitative data were relevant to the tribal community.

Results

Quantitative findings

Of the 12 parents participating in the baseline and follow-up surveys, 33% were male, 92% completed a high school education, 50% were married, and the majority (>50%) were older than 40 years of age. Two of the parents had multiple children who participated in the intervention. Among the 17 youth participating in both surveys, 52.9% were female, the majority were ≥16 years of age, 76.5% were from the community in which the pilot intervention took place, and 82.4% identified as heterosexual (Table 3).

Among the parents, there was an overall increase from 3.3 at baseline in self-evaluated ease in communicating with child about sex (beta = 0.75, SE = 0.27, p = .005). Notable increases in communicating with children about condom use were observed following the pilot intervention. Increases were observed in communicating with children about what to do if a partner doesn't want to use a condom (from 41.7% at baseline to 75% at follow-up, McNemar's chi-square = 4.0, p = .046), how to use a condom (from 8.3% at baseline to 36.4% at follow-up, McNemar's chi-square = 3.0, p = .083), and how well condoms can prevent sexually transmitted infections (from 75% at baseline to 100% at follow-up, McNemar's chi-square = 3.0, p = .083) (Contact corresponding author for detailed results).

Youth attitudes regarding a prospective pregnancy moved in various directions relative to the intervention. There was less agreement with the statements: "it would take away my freedom" (beta = −0.47, SE = 0.2, p = .047) and "my family would be upset or disappointed" (beta = −0.35, SE = 0.2, p = .107). There were larger increases in agreement with the statements "it would encourage me to keep my job or look for a better job," (beta = 0.47, SE = 0.2, p = .005) "it would fit in with my plans" (beta = 0.29, SE = 0.1, p = .033), and "I would consider it a great gift" (beta = 0.29, SE = 0.2, p = .068) (Contact corresponding author for detailed results).

Table 3. Characteristics of parents and youth participating in the pilot intervention.

Characteristics	N	%
Parents	12	
Gender		
Male	4	33.3%
Female	8	66.7%
Town[a]		
Community #1	2	16.7%
Community #2	10	83.3%
Education		
Did not complete high school	1	8.3%
Completed high school	11	91.7%
Marital status		
Married	6	50.0%
Single	3	25.0%
Living with a partner/boyfriend/girlfriend	3	25.0%
Age		
20–30	1	8.3%
31–40	2	16.7%
41–50	6	50.0%
51–60	2	16.7%
61+	1	8.3%
Youth	17	
Gender		
Male	8	47.1%
Female	9	52.9%
Age		
14	1	5.9%
15	1	5.9%
16	7	41.2%
17	3	17.7%
18	4	23.5%
19+	1	5.9%
Town[a]		
Community #1	3	17.7%
Community #2	13	76.5%
Community #3	1	5.9%
Grade level		
9th	3	17.7%
10th	7	41.2%
11th	2	11.8%
12th	5	29.4%
Sexual identification		
Straight/heterosexual	14	82.4%
Bisexual	3	17.7%

[a]The pilot intervention took place in one town on the reservation (Community 2). The majority of the participants came from that town (Community 2) with the remaining participants coming from outside the town (Community 1 and Community 3).

Increases in condom-use self-efficacy were observed across all items (Table 4). Items with larger effect sizes included confidence in one's ability to discuss using condoms with a partner (beta = 0.76, SE = 0.32, p = .016), using a condom with a partner after drinking (beta = 0.54, SE = 0.28, p = .053), and suggesting to use a condom even if there was fear that the partner would think you have an STD (beta = 0.68, SE = 0.36, p = .061).

There was an increase in the ratio of condom use to sexual engagement following the intervention (beta = 0.40, SE = 0.20, p = .05) after controlling for the potentially confounding effects of gender and grade level (see Table 5, Model 1). The direction of the effect remained after controlling for depression and substance use measures, despite a modest reduction in the effect size (beta = 0.31, SE = 0.19, p = .106) (Table 5).

Table 4. Self-efficacy outcomes among youth participating in the pilot intervention, n = 17.

	Unadjusted values				Random intercepts model[a]			
	Pre-intervention		Post-intervention					
How confident … [b]	Mean	SD	Mean	SD	Constant (pre)	SD youth	Beta (post)	(SE)
are you that you could suggest using a condom even if you were afraid that your partner would reject you	3.4	(1.4)	3.3	(1.3)	3.4	0.33	−0.07	0.41
are you that you could suggest using a condom even if you were unsure of how your partner felt about condoms	3.2	(1.3)	3.5	(1.2)	3.2	0.60	0.23	0.32
are you that you could suggest using a condom even if you were afraid that your partner would think that you have had sex with another person before	2.8	(1.2)	3.3	(1.1)	2.8	0.18	0.50	0.37
are you that you could suggest using a condom even if you were afraid that your partner would think you have an STD	2.9	(1.4)	3.6	(1.)	3.0	0.35	0.68	0.36
do you feel in your ability to discuss using condoms with your partner	2.6	(1.4)	3.4	(1.2)	2.6	0.73	0.76	0.32
do you feel in your ability to use a condom correctly	3.1	(1.5)	3.5	(1.1)	3.1	0.91	0.41	0.28
do you feel in your ability to put a condom on without breaking the sexual mood with your partner	2.5	(1.5)	3.2	(1.4)	2.5	0.37	0.66	0.44
do you feel in your ability to buy condoms without feeling embarrassed	2.3	(1.3)	2.8	(1.4)	2.3	1.10	0.47	0.28
are you that you could remember to carry a condom with you in case you need one	2.4	(1.4)	2.9	(1.1)	2.4	0.67	0.56	0.32
do you feel in your ability to use a condom with your partner even after drinking	2.6	(1.5)	3.2	(1.2)	2.6	1.03	0.54	0.28
do you feel in your ability to use a condom with your partner even if you are high	2.6	(1.5)	2.9	(1.2)	2.7	0.54	0.28	0.39
do you feel in your ability to use a condom with your partner even if you are sexually excited	2.9	(1.6)	3.4	(1.3)	3.0	0.79	0.37	0.38

Abbreviations: SE Standard error
[a]Scores have been adjusted for clustering by youth (random intercepts model).
[b]Individual item response sets were 1 = Not at all confident, 2 = Slightly confident, 3 = Moderately confident, 4 = Very confident, 5 = Extremely confident

Table 5. Condom use ratio (# times condom used/# times had sex) relative to depression and substance use in random intercepts models[a] among youth participating in the intervention, n = 17.

	Model 1		Model 2		Model 3		Model 4	
Covariates	Beta	SE	Beta	SE	Beta	SE	Beta	SE
Constant	−0.10	0.62	0.11	0.56	0.08	0.68	0.20	0.57
Gender (male is comparison)	0.17	0.26	0.27	0.24	0.15	0.28	−0.03	0.25
Grade level	0.03	0.12	−0.03	0.11	0.00	0.13	−0.02	0.11
Depression Score	–	–	–	–	0.00	0.02	−0.02	0.02
Number of substances used in the past 30 days			0.18	0.09	–	–	0.24	0.11
Intervention effect	0.40	0.20	0.31	0.18	0.31	0.21	0.31	0.19
SD (youth)	0.08	0.08	0.06	0.05	0.10	0.09	0.06	0.05

Abbreviations: SE Standard error
[a]Scores have been adjusted for clustering by youth (random intercepts model).

Qualitative findings

The primary theme that emerged from the focus groups addressed improved communication. Parents reported improved communication in the following areas: 1) feeling more comfortable talking with their child about SRH because they had talking strategies and techniques after participating in the pilot intervention; 2) more communication within the parent dyad about SRH topics and how as parents they could speak with their child about SRH; 3) awareness of how their own upbringing impacted how they communicate with their child about SRH; and 4) being more comfortable to take their child to Indian Health Services or another clinic for STI testing or birth control.

For youth, improved communication was reported as: 1) feeling less awkward to talk to their parents about SRH; 2) increased understanding of the importance of knowing your family's kinship network and genealogy in order to avoid having an intimate relationship with "a cousin"; 3) feeling more comfortable talking to elders about cultural topics related to SRH; and 4) understanding different ways to communicate with a sex partner other than having sex.

Also addressed in the focus groups were design comments related to the strengths of the pilot intervention as well as possible improvements. Youth identified several benefits to *Native Stand*, including, the inclusivity of LGBTQ issues, a helpful glossary of SRH terms, trustworthy facilitators, and useful SRH lessons. Youth suggested that the pilot intervention be accessible throughout the reservation for course credit. Areas for improvement included: 1) organizing the Native Stand booklet better to reduce redundancies in the information; and 2) increasing the number of learning activities and games that could reinforce key lessons learned during each module.

Parents commented that some of the cultural components presented in *Native Voices* were not relevant to all the tribal members on the reservation because although there are two main tribes living on the reservation, each family may choose to teach their children different cultural ways. Also parents commented that not all families on the reservation practice traditional culture so it would be important in future implementations of the intervention to address contemporary reservation culture in addition to traditional cultural practices related to SRH. Parents reiterated that the parental component of the pilot intervention (*Native Voices*) was beneficial if parents invest time into it. There were suggestions that perhaps an aunt or uncle may be a better guardian/role if the primary parent is unable to attend the *Native Voices* lessons. Parents described wanting more activities that could be used to initiate or maintain conversations with youth. Parents also described wanting more exposure to the materials that youth were receiving during *Native Stand* and the Cultural Mentoring Program.

Discussion and conclusion

The preliminary results from our pilot intervention demonstrate improved SRH outcomes in tribal communities when intervention elements focus on individual, familial, and community level factors. The outcome that appeared to have the greatest impact on sex was increasing parent-child communication. Parents and youth reported more comfort talking about sensitive topics related to sex post participation in our pilot intervention. Specifically parents reported increase in SRH knowledge, in particular knowledge about STIs, birth control, how to use a condom, increased strategies for speaking with youth about sex, and increased communication within their parent dyad relationship.

There are several implications to these findings. Simply because one is a parent does not mean that they know about different SRH topics or that they are comfortable talking with their children about sex. Our pilot intervention suggests the importance of providing parents with similar education as their children. The need to provide parents with SRH education may be particularly important within AI families because of cultural norms regarding who can speak with whom within a family about SRH as well as the legacy of sexual violence and trauma within AI families, which may make it awkward and difficult to talk about SRH. Reported increased engagement in intrafamilial communication between parent dyads in our pilot intervention is also promising.

These findings highlight the need to rebuild traditional pathways of communication about SRH within AI families. Traditionally topics related to SRH were passed down in families and kinship networks through grandparents, aunts and uncles either in private conversations or through ceremonies. This communication pathway and teaching mechanism were disrupted through children being forced to leave home to be raised in boarding schools, forbidden to practice their traditional ceremonies or speak their Native language (Bigfoot & Funderburk, 2011). Parent education programs that provide knowledge to parents about SRH topics and how to communicate about SRH can have a positive impact on strengthening and healing AI families from the SRH injustices that created the context for the SRH disparities in today's AI communities (White et al., 2006).

Youths' attitudes toward pregnancy demonstrated that pregnancy would not take away their freedom or create discord within their family. Youth also reported that pregnancy: 1) had a positive influence on their motivations to get a good job; 2) fit into their life plans; and 3) was a gift. Previous research on attitudes toward pregnancy and pregnancy dynamics in AI communities demonstrate that pregnancy is central to traditional and cultural beliefs about the sacredness of life, the continuation of family and sacred knowledge, and essential to the continuation of a tribe, clan or band of people. Historically, pregnancy prevention interventions with AI populations have promoted colonial, predominately Christian beliefs about pregnancy such as waiting to have children until marriage, completion of post-secondary education and job/financial security (Hagen et al., 2012; McMahon et al., 2015). These colonial Christian based values do not always resonate with AI communities and do not adequately take into account the history of cultural and structural violence perpetrated on AI communities, which have contributed to poor SRH outcomes among AIs. From a Christian based pregnancy prevention paradigm, the attitudes toward pregnancy expressed by the youth in our pilot intervention could be viewed as troublesome because the results indicate that pregnancy is a positive part of a youth's life and is not viewed as a barrier to achieving life goals. From an AI viewpoint our pilot intervention results resonate with cultural beliefs and values regarding pregnancy and suggest the need to decolonize attitudes toward pregnancy that are based on colonial, Christian ideals (Gurr, 2012).

Youth self-reported increases in condom use self-efficacy, condom negotiation skills with a partner while drinking, and understanding STI risks. These findings reinforce the importance of integrating SRH education into educational systems as a standard of practice. Youth demonstrated an increase in condom use during sex after participating in the pilot intervention, regardless of gender or age. Increased condom use during sex also held true after considering depression and substance use. These findings hold promise despite the small effect size and lack of statistical significant. Empowering youth to take responsibility for their choices can begin to reconstruct AI youth's concepts of bodily determination that were eroded during Colonialization as a result of policies aimed at undermining AI peoples' decisions about their reproduction (Lumsden, 2016).

The feedback from the parents and youth in our focus groups suggested positive impacts of the pilot intervention and constructive suggestions for improvements. For example, SRH educational support for parents while their children are in high school may be helpful. Parents also suggested that including extended family such as aunts or uncles in the parent component of our intervention would be useful if parents are not able to attend. Youth feedback demonstrated the importance of strengthening intergenerational communication about cultural beliefs and practices related to SRH. This suggestion demonstrates the importance of extended family involvement in AI communities in which kinship relationships beyond the nuclear family are integral to family functioning. The integration of extended family members in interventions for AI communities supports traditional practices within families in which aunts, uncles and grandparents participated in the raising of children (Hossain et al., 2011; Hungry Wolf, 1982).

Our study had limitations. We used validated measures in our study. We also used CASI to increase perceived privacy and mitigate social desirability bias (Ghanem et al., 2005). However, because of our limited sample size for youth and parents our effect sizes were small and warrant cautious interpretation despite the reliability of the measures we used and our computerized data collection method. We conducted two focus groups which may not have gleaned feedback that was reflective of all youth and parents that participated in our pilot intervention. Although cultural adaptations were made to the *Native Stand* and *Native Voices* curricula, culturally specificity may hinder applicable to other tribes in different cultural contexts. Our pilot intervention did not include a system's level that addressed the coordination and access of SRH services for youth on the reservation. Previous research has documented the challenges of SRH services for AIs, such as accessibility, cultural appropriateness, and mistrust of health care providers (De Ravello et al., 2012). A system's level component may have strengthened our pilot intervention.

In summary, the purpose of this manuscript was to present the findings from a pilot intervention for AI youth and their parents aimed at reducing SRH disparities. Our results provide evidence for the positive impact a multi-level, multi-component intervention has for: 1) increasing knowledge and skills necessary to reduce high risk sexual behavior which can lead to poor SRH outcomes in tribal communities; and 2) increasing intrafamilial and intergenerational communication about SRH topics. Our pilot intervention supports the need for tribally tailored SRH interventions for youth and families. In order to improve SRH outcomes that have plagued AI communities since the onset of Colonialization innovative multi-level interventions must be developed, implemented and evaluated. Future research is needed to test the efficacy of multi-level, multi-component tribally driven SRH interventions for AI youth and their families that integrate contemporary realities of SRH issues with traditional values and beliefs.

Acknowledgments

The tribally based research team and the university based research team would like to thank the school administrators, teachers, youth and parents who participated in the pilot intervention, the elders who worked with us on the pilot intervention as well as the members of our study's community advisory board. Their respective participation was central to the important knowledge gained from our pilot intervention.

Disclosure statement

No potential conflict of interest was reported by the authors.

Funding

This work was supported by the Center for American Indian and Rural Health Equity (CAIRHE) at Montana State University through the National Institute of General Medical Sciences Award Number : P20GM104417.

References

Arnold, S. B. (2014). Reproductive rights denied: The Hyde Amendment and access to abortion for Native American women using Indian health service facilities. *American Journal of Public Health*, *104*(10), 1892–1893. https://doi.org/10.2105/AJPH.2014.302084

ATLAS.ti Scientific Software Development GmbH. Version 7.5.16.GmbH, Berlin. http://atlasti.com. 2020.

Beckett, M. K., Elliott, M. N., Martino, S., Kanouse, D. E., Corona, R., Klein, D. J., & Schuster, M. A. (2010). Timing of parent and child communication about sexuality relative to children's sexual behaviors. *Pediatrics*, *125*(1), 34–42. https://doi.org/10.1542/peds.2009-0806

Beckman, L. J., Harvey, S. M., & Murray, J. (1992). Dimensions of the contraceptive attributes questionnaire. *Psychology of Women Quarterly*, *16*(2), 243–259. https://doi.org/10.1111/j.1471-6402.1992.tb00253.x

Bernstein, E., Ashong, D., Heeren, T., Winter, M., Bliss, C., Madico, G., & Bernstein, J. (2012). The impact of a brief motivational intervention on unprotected sex and sex while high among drug-positive emergency department patients who receive STI/HIV VC/T and drug treatment referral as standard of care. *AIDS and Behavior*, *16*(5), 1203–1216. https://doi.org/10.1007/s10461-012-0134-0

Bigfoot, D., & Funderburk, B. (2011). Honoring children, making relatives: The cultural translation of parent-child interaction therapy for American Indian and Alaska Native families. *Journal of Psychoactive Drugs*, *43*(4), 309–318. https://doi.org/10.1080/02791072.2011.628924

Bronfenbrenner, U. (1999). Environments in developmental perspective: Theoretical and operational models. In S. L. Friedman & T. D. Wachs (Eds.), *Measuring environment across the life span: Emerging methods and concepts* (pp. 3–28). American Psychological Association.

Centers for Disease Control and Prevention. (2013). *U.S. Teen pregnancy outcomes by age, race and hispanic ethnicity*. https://www.cdc.gov/teenpregnancy/pdf/teen-pregnancy-rates-2013.pdf

Centers for Disease Control and Prevention. (2014). *Health disparities in HIV/AIDS, Virtal Hepatitis, STDs, and TB American Indians/Alaska Natives*. https://www.cdc.gov/nchhstp/healthdisparities/americanindians.html

Centers for Disease Control and Prevention. (2017a). *HIV among American Indians and Alaska Natives in the United States*. https://www.cdc.gov/hiv/group/racialethnic/aian/index.html

Centers for Disease Control and Prevention. (2017b). *Youth risk behavior survey*. https://www.cdc.gov/healthyyouth/data/yrbs/questionnaires.htm

Corbin, J., & Strauss, A. (2008). *Basics of qualitative research: Techniques and procedures for developing grounded theory.* SAGE Publications.

De Ravello, L., Everett Jones, S., Tulloch, S., Taylor, M., & Doshi, S. (2014). Substance use and sexual risk behaviors among American Indian and Alaska Native high school students. *Journal of School Health, 84*(1), 25–32. https://doi.org/10.1111/josh.12114

De Ravello, L., Tulloch, S., & Taylor, M. (2012). We will be known forever by the tracks we leave: Rising up to meet the reproductive health needs of American Indian and Alaska Native youth. *American Indian and Alaska Native Mental Health Research, (Online), 19*(1), i. https://doi.org/10.5820/aian.1901.2012.i

Ghanem, K. G., Hutton, H. E., Zenilman, J. M., Zimba, R., & Erbelding, E. J. (2005). Audio computer assisted self interview and face to face interview modes in assessing response bias among STD clinic patients. *Sexually Transmitted Infections, 81*(5), 421. https://doi.org/10.1136/sti.2004.013193

Gurr, B. (2012). The failures and possibilities of a human rights approach to secure Native American women's reproductive justice. *Societies Without Borders, 7*(1), 1–28.

Hagen, J. W., Skenandore, A. H., Scow, B. M., Schanen, J. G., & Clary, F. H. (2012). Adolescent pregnancy prevention in a rural Native American community. *Journal of Family Social Work, 15*(1), 19–33. https://doi.org/10.1080/10522158.2012.640926

Hanson, J. D., McMahon, T. R., Griese, E. R., & Kenyon, D. B. (2014). Understanding gender roles in teen pregnancy prevention among American Indian youth. *American Journal of Health Behavior, 38*(6), 807–815. https://doi.org/10.5993/AJHB.38.6.2

Haroz, E. E., Ybarra, M. L., & Eaton, W. W. (2014). Psychometric evaluation of a self-report scale to measure adolescent depression: The CESDR-10 in two national adolescent samples in the United States. *Journal of Affective Disorders, 158*, 154–160. https://doi.org/10.1016/j.jad.2014.02.009

Hossain, Z., Skurky, T., Joe, J., & Hunt, T. (2011). The sense of collectivism and individualism among husbands and wives in traditional and bi-cultural Navajo Indian families on the Navajo reservation. *Journal of Comparative Family Studies, 42*(4), 543–562. https://doi.org/10.3138/jcfs.42.4.543

Hungry Wolf, B. (1982). *The ways of my grandmothers* (1st Quill ed.). Quill.

Jerman, P., & Constantine, N. A. (2010). Demographic and psychological predictors of parent–adolescent communication about sex: A representative statewide analysis. *Journal of Youth and Adolescence, 39*(10), 1164–1174. https://doi.org/10.1007/s10964-010-9546-1

Lumsden, S. (2016). Reproductive justice, sovereignity & incarceration: Prison abolition politics & California Indians. *American Indian Culture and Research Journal, 40*(1), 1. https://doi.org/10.17953/aicrj.40.1.lumsden

McMahon, T. R., Hanson, J. D., Griese, E. R., & Kenyon, D. B. (2015). Teen pregnancy prevention program recommendations from urban and reservation northern plains American Indian community members. *American Journal of Sexuality Education, 10*(3), 218–241. https://doi.org/10.1080/15546128.2015.1049314

Mitchell, C., Keane, E., Yazzie, L., Cottier, N., & Crow, C. B. (2000). *Pathways of choice survey.* http://www.ucdenver.edu/academics/colleges/PublicHealth/research/centers/CAIANH/NCAIANMHR/ResearchProjects/Documents/choicsrv.pdf

Rink, E., Bird, E. A. R., Fourstar, K., Ricker, A., Runs-Above, W., Meyers, A. A., & Hallum-Montes, R. (2016). Partnering with American Indian communities in strength-based collaborative health research: Guiding principles from the Fort Peck ceremony of research project. *American Indian and Alaska Native Mental Health Research, 23*(3), 187. https://doi.org/10.5820/aian.2303.2016.187

StataCorp. (2015). *Stata 14.1.* Stata Corporation.

Tingey, L., Chambers, R., Goklish, N., Larzelere, F., Lee, A., Suttle, R., Rosenstock, S., Lake, K., & Barlow, A. (2017). Rigorous evaluation of a pregnancy prevention program for American Indian youth and adolescents: Tudy protocol for a randomized controlled trial. *Trials, 18*(1), 89. https://doi.org/10.1186/s13063-017-1842-6

White, J., Godfrey, J., & Iron Mocassin, B. (2006). American Indian fathering in the Dakota Nation: Use of Akicita as a fatherhood standard. *Fathering A Journal of Theory, Research, and Practice about Men as Fathers, 4*(1), 49–69. https://doi.org/10.3149/fth.0401.49

Whitesell, N., Asdigian, N., Kaufman, C., Big Crow, C., Shangreau, C., Keane, E., Mousseau, A. C., & Mitchell, C. (2014). Trajectories of substance use among young American Indian adolescents: Patterns and predictors. *Journal of Youth and Adolescence, 43*(3), 437–453. https://doi.org/10.1007/s10964-013-0026-2

SACRED Connections: A university-tribal clinical research partnership for school-based screening and brief intervention for substance use problems among Native American youth

Staci L. Morris, Michelle M. Hospital, Eric F. Wagner, John Lowe, Michelle G. Thompson, Rachel Clarke, and Cheryl Riggs

ABSTRACT

Native American (NA) youth report higher rates of alcohol, marijuana, and drug use than U.S. adolescents from any other racial/ethnic group. Addressing this health disparity is a significant research priority across public health, minority health, and dissemination and implementation (D&I) sciences, underscoring the need for empirically-based interventions tailored for NA youth. Effective D&I with NA youth incorporates NA cultural values and involves tribal elders and stakeholders. SACRED Connections (NIDA R01DA02977) was a university-tribal research partnership that utilized a culturally derived Native-Reliance theoretical framework and a community-based participatory research (CBPR) approach. A significant objective of this randomized controlled trial was to close D&I gaps utilizing the RE-AIM Model and National Culturally and Linguistically Appropriate Services (CLAS) in Health and Health Care Standards (HHS, 2019).

Findings of this 5-year RCT revealed a statistically significant protective relationship between Native Reliance and baseline lifetime and past month alcohol and marijuana use; additionally, the likelihood of reporting marijuana use at 3 months post-intervention was significantly lower among the active condition than among the control condition. Implementation of a developmentally and NA culturally tailored brief protocol revealed: partnering with Native Americans and utilizing CBPR facilitated engagement with this hard-to-reach, underserved community; age and culture are associated with substance use severity among NA teens; a culturally adapted Motivational Interviewing (MI) brief intervention may be effective in reducing marijuana use among NA youth; the Native Reliance theory proved useful as a framework for working with this population; and RE-AIM proved helpful in conceptualizing health equity promoting D&I.

Substance use among Native American (NA) youth

Native Americans (NA) experience disproportionately high rates of substance use problems, yet data suggest that many do not receive effective interventions to manage substance use and associated comorbid conditions. Incidence rates for accidental death, domestic violence, suicide, incarceration, illness, and disease associated with substance use among NA people are between 2–3.5 times higher than any other ethnic group (Baciu et al., 2017; Center for Behavioral Health Statistics and Quality (CBHSQ), SAMHSA & US HHS, 2011; Urban Indian Health Institute (UIHI), 2011, 2014a). Incidence rates per 100,000 NA persons for alcohol and illicit drug use disorders among NA people age 12 and older are higher than any other US racial/ethnic group (Center for Behavioral Health Statistics and Quality (CBHSQ), SAMHSA & US HHS, 2011). Furthermore, NA mortality rates per 100,000 NA persons, compared with the general U.S. population, are markedly elevated for alcohol related liver disease/cirrhosis (21.6% vs. 9.2%), and alcohol induced death (11.7% vs. 3.3%) (Centers for Disease Control and Prevention (CDC), 2014). This health disparity plaguing NA people is a product of social exclusion, discrimination, poverty, historical trauma, and the disregard for NA cultural values that affect stress proliferation (Pearlin et al., 1997); these factors influence health-care decisions which can lead to maladaptive behaviors, substance use problems, and psychosocial vulnerability (Brave Heart, 1999; Brave Heart & DeBruyn, 1998; Lowe et al., 2016; Snijder et al., 2018).

NA teenagers are at particularly high risk for substance use and substance use problems compared to teenagers from any other racial/ethnic group. NA youth report higher rates of past month cigarette use, binge drinking, and illicit drug use compared to U.S. adolescents from any other racial/ethnic group (SAMHSA, 2004; Snijder et al., 2018). NA adolescents tend to start using earlier and have more severe consequences, including higher rates of suicide and loss of potential years of life (e.g., Bachman et al., 1991; Beauvais, 1996; Center for Behavioral Health Statistics and Quality (CBHSQ), SAMHSA & US HHS, 2011; Burnette & Figley, 2016; Gfellner & Hundleby, 1995; Gutierres et al., 1994; Guttmannova et al., 2017; Substance Abuse and Mental Health Services Administration (SAMHSA), 2004, 2008; Schinke et al., 2000; UIHI, 2014a). According to the National Survey on Drug Use and Health, nearly 9.2% of NA ages 12 and older reported current heavy alcohol use, the highest rate of any ethnic group (Substance Abuse and Mental Health Services Administration (SAMHSA), 2015). Moreover, NA youth ages 12–17 reported twice the rate of past month marijuana use than non-Hispanics Whites (14.6% v. 7.1%) (Substance Abuse and Mental Health Services Administration (SAMHSA), 2019).

Adolescence is a crucial period within which to intervene as it is a key period of brain development that can be severely negatively impacted by early and heavy alcohol and other substance use (Morris & Wagner, 2007). Since NA youth are at especially high risk for substance use, developing effective interventions for NA teenagers is a significant research priority. Guttmannova et al. (2017) suggest that despite the reported differences in initiation and rates of alcohol and substance use, the trends among all US teenagers are similar; therefore, rather than reinventing a specific NA intervention, they suggest culturally adapting evidence-based interventions for use with NA youth.

Motivational interviewing

Motivational Interviewing (MI; Arkowitz et al., 2015) is an evidence-based, directive, client-centered, collaborative counseling style. MI enhances motivation for change by helping the client clarify and resolve ambivalence about behavior change, thereby creating cognitive dissonance between where one is now and where one wants to be. A consistent empirical literature supports the effectiveness of motivational interviewing (MI) with adolescent substance users. While there are over two decades of published reports of randomized clinical trials (RCT's) of MI with adolescent alcohol and marijuana users demonstrating its effectiveness (Borsari & Carey, 2000; D'Amico et al., 2008, 2018; Daeppen et al., 2011; Larimer et al., 2001; Martin et al., 2005; McCambridge & Strang, 2004, 2005; Monti et al., 1999; Newton et al., 2018; Roberts et al., 2000; Stein et al., 2006; Walker et al., 2006), studies of MI with NA youth have been limited (Wagner et al., in press). The consequences of health disparities, such as lack of funding, private space in small schools, institutional barriers, poverty, etc. are recognized as barriers to implementation. The current study was a D&I effort to address this problem and overcome identified barriers in an underserved population (Native Americans).

The underpinnings of motivational interviewing are consistent with Native Americans beliefs (D.L. Dickerson et al., 2016; Gilder et al., 2011; Venner et al., 2007). In their study utilizing a culturally adapted version of MI with American Indian/Alaska Native youth, D.L. Dickerson et al. (2016) reported that "urban AI/AN youth liked the open and collaborative nature of MI and said that this approach helped them feel more connected with each other." Batliner et al. (2014) stressed that access to services for Native Americans is limited by virtue of high poverty rates, their rural location, and corresponding lack of treatment facilities, rendering them a medically underserved population; this is further complicated by the fact that while effective, brief interventions by virtue of the limited time for relationship building may prohibit the development of trust with a group who is distrustful of outsiders. These barriers and obstacles were addressed in the current study.

Approach

A community-based participatory research (CBPR) approach was utilized following principles that guided a partnered approach in all phases of the research process. This ensured equitable involvement by community members, academic researchers, and others (such as the Health Educators who conducted the MI sessions) and solidified the research partnership. All partners contributed expertise and shared in decision making and ownership of the project (Israel et al., 2003; Wallerstein & Duran, 2003). Following this CBPR approach allowed the joining of the health research team and tribal community members, which resulted in a genuine voice in the research process and the intervention's successful implementation and attainment of project goals (Wallerstein & Duran, 2010).

Method

Purpose

SACRED Connections (Self-Awareness Creates Responsible Empowered Decisions) was a 5-year RCT (NIDA R01DA02977, PI: Wagner) that formed an effective university-community partnership to culturally adapt, implement, and evaluate a brief evidence-based motivational substance use intervention among NA youth in Midwestern rural communities. Essential to the success of the project was the guidance received by school administrators, a prominent tribal chief, and a local Community Advisory Board (CAB). The primary goal of the proposed study was to conduct a clinical trial evaluating a culturally congruent, school-based motivational interviewing intervention targeting substance use among NA high school students. The study had 4 aims:

Aim #1: To compare three intervention conditions: (1) Brief Advice and a Personalized Feedback Report alone (BA+PFR; n = 160), (2) Brief Advice, a Personalized Feedback Report, and Motivational Interviewing (BA+PFR+MI; n = 160), and (3) Brief Advice, a Personalized Feedback Report, Motivational Interviewing, and a 6-months post-intervention Booster session (BA+PFR+MI +BOOST; n = 160).

Aim #2: To evaluate the impact of a 6-months-post-intervention booster session on substance use and substance-related negative consequences.

Aim #3: To examine putative mechanisms of change (i.e., mediators) associated with response to our motivational interviewing intervention.

Aim #4: To explore gender and Native American cultural variables as moderators of intervention response.

Measures

As seen in Figure 1, all participants were evaluated at study entry (baseline), and at 3-, 6-, 9-, and 12-month follow-ups. The baseline interview took approximately 1 hour to complete; each follow-up assessment took approximately 30 minutes to complete. All assessment measures were carefully selected based on reliability, validity, developmental and cultural appropriateness and were approved by the CAB. Screening was conducted using The Personal Experience Screening Questionnaire (PESQ; Winters, 1991), designed to identify adolescents in need of a substance use assessment and referral. The use of screenings has been suggested by the Urban Indian Health Institute (Urban Indian Health Institute, 2014b) to overcome barriers to access and improve treatment outcomes. The PESQ takes

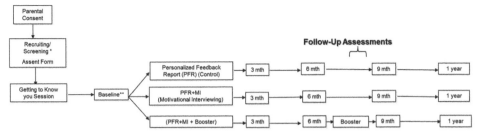

Figure 1. Participant flow chart.
*participants were recruited from 6 rural public high schools across 2 counties
**random assignment of condition

approximately 10 minutes to complete. Demographic information and counseling history were assessed as well as:

Substance Use Disorder Diagnosis: The Composite International Diagnostic Interview (CIDI), developed by the World Health Organization (WHO), is a comprehensive, fully structured diagnostic interview, designed to be administered by lay interviewers and was a product of more than 15 years of international collaboration aimed at standardized procedures for assessing disorders in community studies throughout the world (Kessler et al., 1998).

Substance Use Patterns: Substance use at each contact was measured using the Timeline Followback Interview (TLFB; Sobell & Sobell, 1992, 1996; Sobell et al., 1980). Substance consumption information was collected using a calendar format to provide temporal cues (e.g., holidays, special occurrences) to assist in recall of days when substances were used. Alcohol use was measured in standard drinks and substance use was collected in terms of use/nonuse given wide variations in potency and ingestion methods. Additionally, 10% of participants were randomly selected at both the 6-month and 12-month follow-up assessments for urine testing using the OnTrak TesTcup® (4 Panel) from Varian Diagnostics (http://www.varianinc.com/cgi-bin/nav?/products/dat/testcup).

Substance Use Consequences were assessed using The Drug Use Screening Inventory-Revised (DUSI-R; Tarter, 1990), a multidimensional questionnaire concerning teenager's alcohol, marijuana, and other drug use frequency, substance use problem severity, and related domains (e.g., school performance, health status, peer relationships).

Readiness to change was assessed using a readiness ruler (Rollnick et al., 1999) on a continuum from *not ready to change* (0) to *trying to change* (10). A similar measure was used to assess the importance of changing substance use from *not important at all* (0) to *the most important thing in my life* (100).

Self-efficacy to resist substance use was measured via The Brief Situational Confidence Questionnaire (BSCQ), an 8-item version of the 39-item SCQ (Annis & Graham, 1988) that covers eight areas of high-risk situations for relapse in the SCQ. Respondents rated each situation regarding their confidence to resist urges to use substances, from 1 (*not at all confident*) to 100 (*totally confident*).

Native American Culture was assessed using the Native Reliance Framework (Lowe, 2002; Lowe et al., 2016, 2019). Cultural variables are related to values associated with rural community living. These values are steeped in the culture where the collective or group is emphasized versus individualism. As seen in Figure 2, Native Reliance is a cultural identity theoretical framework that describes the beliefs and values of *seeking truth* and *making connections, being responsible, being disciplined*, and *being confident. Seeking truth and making connections* for NA refers to knowing the spirit in everything, including themselves, so that connections become known in all aspects of their lives. *Being responsible* refers to providing by having an income and also accepting assistance for what is necessary. *Being responsible* refers to individuals learning and accepting the role of caring for the well-being of themselves and others such as family and community members. This may require NA individuals to

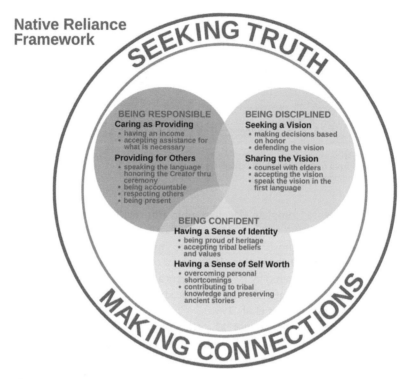

Figure 2. Native reliance.

accept assistance offered by tribal programs or other individuals within their tribal communities. *Being responsible* also refers to providing for others by respecting others, being present and accountable, and by calling on the Creator through speaking the traditional Native/Indigenous language and honoring the Creator through ceremony. *Being disciplined* refers to seeking a vision by making decisions based on honor and defending the vision. *Being disciplined* also refers to sharing the vision by counseling with elders, accepting the vision, and speaking the vision in the traditional Indigenous language. *Being confident* refers to having a sense of identity by being proud of one's Indigenous heritage and accepting Indigenous or tribal beliefs and values. *Being confident* also refers to having a sense of self-worth by facing challenges and contributing to Indigenous or tribal knowledge and preserving ancestral stories. These beliefs and values are arranged in a circular manner to represent the circular nature of an Indigenous world view.

Finally, at the one year follow-up, participants completed the Interventionist Description Form, a version of McLennan's (1990) 12-item Counselor Perception Measure (CPM), adapted for use with substance using youth to measure participants' perceptions of the Health Educator's (project staff) acceptance and competence.

All participants were randomly assigned to one of three treatment conditions: (1) Brief Advice and a Personalized Feedback Report alone (BA+PFR), (2) Brief Advice, a Personalized Feedback Report, and Motivational Interviewing (BA+PFR+MI), or (3) Brief Advice, a Personalized Feedback Report, Motivational Interviewing, and a 6-month post-intervention Booster session (BA+PFR+MI+BOOST). While the Health Educators were aware of condition assignment, participants were blind to condition assignment. The Health Educators were made aware of the nature of randomization during trainings and supervisors were trained to remain vigilant to any differences in the delivery of the intervention.

D&I and the RE-AIM model

The science of D&I guides development, implementation, and dissemination of evidence-based practices while accounting for adaptations through the use of models. Dissemination, implementation, and evaluation of this study were guided by the RE-AIM D&I model (re-aim.org, 2017). The evidence-based practice was Motivational Interviewing (MI). As seen in Figure 3, RE-AIM is a non-linear framework that equally accounts for dissemination and implementation and allows for adaptations during the process. RE-AIM was developed to assist in the development and evaluation of real-world public health programs with the ultimate goal of implementing effective, generalizable, evidence-based interventions. RE-AIM was the model most often used in NIH and CDC D&I grant applications between 2006 and 2016 (Harden et al., 2018; Vinson et al., 2017). As shown in Figure 3 (re-aim.org, 2017), the plan cycles through the 5 key RE-AIM dimensions: (1) Reach; (2) Effectiveness; (3) Adoption; (4) Implementation, and (5) Maintenance. However, RE-AIM phases are best understood in the following order: (1) Adoption, (2) Reach, (3) Implementation, (4) Effectiveness, and (5) Maintenance.

Adoption

Adoption refers to the number and representativeness of entities and interventionists. The key question is, "How can organizational (systemic level) support be developed?" For the current study, this was accomplished in several ways: trainings with Health Educators, the first of which was in Midwestern rural communities where the researchers were immersed in NA culture and traditions; development of the project name and logo guided by NA tribal stakeholders and project staff; continued involvement in traditional NA holidays, parades, and celebrations; annual CAB meetings

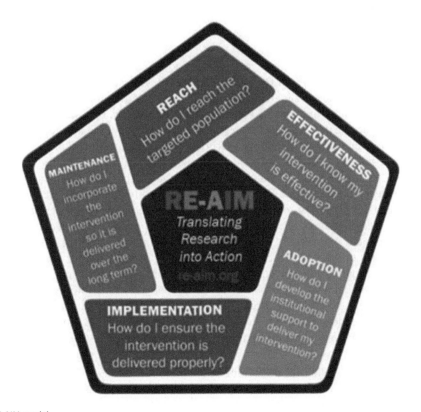

Figure 3. RE-AIM model.
Elements of the RE-AIM Framework (Cummings Graduate Institute (2015–2019), retrieved from https://azhin.org/cummings/re-aim)

with key stakeholders who reviewed and provided feedback on project materials and implementation strategies continually identifying and addressing pathways and barriers to adoption; repeated presentations to tribal leaders and school staff; and obtaining 2 tribal IRB approvals.

In particular, the CAB recommended that key tribal community members with expertise in substance use counseling engage with the HEs and researchers in "mock" sessions using the proposed materials and intervention strategies. During these sessions, the HEs and researchers received feedback and input from the tribal experts. For example, body language, posture, and voice tones that could potentially be considered intrusive, disrespectful, and threatening and may have resulted in the youth participants disengaging in the project sessions were noted by the tribal experts. This CBPR principle is referred to as "participation with action" (Israel et al., 2003) and was a crucial, yet time consuming process. It became apparent that extra training sessions were needed which presented a project challenge as extra training sessions meant additional time and resources, which not only included salaries for project staff, but also compensation for community consultants who dedicated their time and had a cultural expectation of meal provision and shared food, expenses often not covered by grant funding.

The NA youth were located in rural Midwestern communities where resources are limited. The communities are small with long distances separating them from other communities. Therefore, there is great reliance and dependence on each other and many communities comprise multiple related families. Most of the communities are of lower socioeconomic status and the majority of incomes come from labor jobs such as farming and construction. Ultimately, the project was implemented in 6 schools across 2 counties.

Staffing proved to be a crucial component; the project coordinator and Health Educators were tribally enrolled, trained in mental health, and immersed in both Native and school communities. RE-AIM proposes an Adoption calculator which is equal to sites participated/approached. In terms of schools approached, all schools participated, so the Adoption rate was 100% (6/6).

Reach

The total population (REACH) of this 5-year RCT included NA tribal community elders (n = 14), Health Educators (n = 15), and youth (N = 405); total N = 434. Reach accounts for the number and representativeness of participants on an individual level. The key question is, "How can the targeted population be reached on an individual level?" For the current study, this was accomplished by: (1) cultural tailoring regarding the language, images, and references with input and approval by the CAB; (2) repeated meetings and class presentations at schools; and (3) recognition of program participation at holidays and at the end of the school year. CAB members' feedback and approval proved to be crucial to the success of the project, specifically in terms of Reach. CAB members remained active during the entire length of the project. The CAB met regularly throughout the duration of the project and was instrumental in reviewing and approving all materials, receiving updates by the research team on a regular basis regarding the progress of the project, and was provided a report of the findings at the conclusion of the project. Additionally, they provided cultural interpretation regarding the findings of the study. CBPR stresses the importance of cultural tailoring of intervention, acknowledging native and Western science approaches, and supporting the selection of a culturally appropriate framework (D.L. Dickerson et al., 2016; D. Dickerson et al., 2018; Getty, 2010; Whitbeck et al., 2012). CAB meetings allowed for this process to occur, for the materials to be culturally and scientifically appropriate, and their endorsement was pivotal in obtaining consent. This process was informed by The National CLAS (culturally and linguistically appropriate services) Standards (HHS, 2019), 15 action steps intended to ensure heath care for diverse populations is provided in culturally and linguistically sensitive and respectful approaches.

Clinical trial participants were recruited from rural public schools with predominantly NA students by NA project staff who had a consistent presence at the schools for project purposes and important school and NA events and holidays. CAB involvement and endorsement were acknowledged during in-school recruitment presentations. The RE-AIM Reach calculator is equal to # of participants

(N = 405)/# eligible (461), making Reach 87.85%. Reach also accounts for attrition, which was calculated overall and for each assessment time point: Overall attrition (baseline-12 mos) = 259/ 405 = 36%, followed by 15% 3 month attrition, 11.3% 6 month attrition, 15.1% 9 month attrition, and 6.2% 12 month attrition. Reach also considers whether the sample was representative of the population; demographics for this sample were as follows: mean age 16.37 (*SD* 1.26); sex 49.8% female; grade level 9th (14.8%), 10th (25.4%), 11th (30%), and 12th (32.2%). It is important to note that 12th graders were not included in the original recruitment plan due to the 12 month follow-up; however, the CAB urged for inclusiveness so inclusion criteria was altered accordingly.

Implementation

The next phase in the RE-AIM process after the intervention was adopted and participants were reached was implementation. Implementation refers to fidelity to the intervention's protocol. The key questions are: "What activities are required?" and "Is the protocol being implemented as intended?" This was accomplished through (1) the development of the protocol and manuals, which included cultural tailoring; (2) securing of confidential locations; (3) determining who would deliver the intervention and initial and subsequent trainings at least twice a year at the beginning and end of each school year; and (4) supervision, which included weekly reports, monthly video calls, and tracking of project achievements and problematic activities.

For the current study, inclusion criteria for the substance use screening were: (1) 9th, 10th, 11th or 12th grade enrollment; (2) self-reported NA race/ethnicity; (3) active parental consent; and (4) student assent. The intervention phase of the clinical trial had the added inclusion criterion "substance user," operationalized as the use of drugs or alcohol on one or more occasions during the past 90-days. Exclusion criteria for the intervention were: (1) clinically significant mental health problems (e.g., depression) as identified through assessment and interview; (2) clinically significant substance use problems as identified through assessment and interview; or, (3) behavior that places the participant or others around him in danger (e.g., suicidality).

Prior to initiating the screening assessment, written parental consent was obtained. Adolescent participants' informed assent was obtained by project staff prior to taking part in the screening and clinical phases of the study. In response to feedback from Health Educators, a rapport building "getting to know you" initial meeting with participants was added prior to conducting the baseline assessment in order for participants to feel comfortable disclosing accurate reports of their substance use at the next meeting. During this meeting, Health Educators met with participants and discussed: the description of the program and topics addressed; the assessment schedule and types of questions to be asked; confidentiality; planning for a convenient time for the baseline assessment and personalized feedback session; and any questions or concerns.

All clinical trial participants (overall N = 480) completed a baseline assessment, and were randomly assigned to one of three treatment conditions: (1) BA+PFR; n = 160, (2) BA+PFR+MI; n = 160, or (3) BA+PFR+MI+BOOST; n = 160. BA+PFR involved a meeting with a Health Educator during which participants were given an informational handout about the risks of drug and alcohol use, a list of local substance abuse treatment resources, and their own personalized feedback report (PFR).In addition, BA+PFR participants were encouraged to stop using substances and to get assistance if necessary. Both BA+PFR+MI and BA+PFR+MI+BOOST participants took part in a motivational interview feedback session, which (a) was conducted based on the techniques of MI (Miller & Rollnick, 1991, 2002) and (b) included written personalized feedback in areas including descriptive norms, perceived beliefs regarding friends' and parents' approval of drug and alcohol use, financial costs of drug and alcohol use, and self-reported negative consequences of substance use. Also discussed were the participant's typical use patterns, social supports for reducing or ending use, personal goals and their relation to substance use, and how important and confident the teen was about reducing substance use.

The PFR was a computer generated personalized intervention booklet that utilized participant reported substance use from the baseline assessment. The resulting booklet was printed in color and presented much of the feedback and intervention activities graphically in order to be engaging and consistent with motivational strategies. It contained a summary of age at first alcohol and marijuana use and lifetime alcohol and marijuana use as well as comparative rates of other adolescents in the same state. This allowed for examination of patterns of use as well as focusing in on consequences of substance use. There was a section on confidence to resist substance use in various situations, set goals, consider social support, and a change plan on how to reduce substance use and anticipate possible barriers. At the 12-month follow-up assesment, 89 participants completed a Participant Feedback Report; 92% reported that they liked the materials used.

After the 6-month follow-up assessment, BA+PFR+MI+BOOST participants received a MI booster session; the format paralleled that used in the initial MI intervention with personalized feedback provided in the areas of self-reported substance use, self-reported substance use problems, perceived current and future risks of substance use, impact of substance use on short- and long-term personal goals, social support for making changes in substance use patterns, and methods for risk reduction. The booster session also included feedback about changes in use patterns based on data collected at baseline, 3-month, and 6-month assessments. The only difference between BA+PFR+MI participants and BA+PFR+MI+BOOST participants was whether or not they received a booster session at 6-months post-intervention.

Participants were evaluated at study entry (baseline), and at 3-, 6-, 9-, and 12-month follow-ups. Assessments addressed demographic and background variables, drug and alcohol use, drug and alcohol use-related problems, and indicators of Native American cultural variables. To aid in participant retention, all research participants received gift cards of increasing value over time ranging from 20 USD to 50, USD resulting in a potential remuneration of 160 USD for complete participation through the 12 month follow-up.

As far as measurement of implementation, RE-AIM does not propose an implementation calculator, but rather recommends accounting for consistency of implementation or the extent to which protocol was implemented as intended, while acknowledging that unfortunately, such data are hardly ever available. Fidelity to implementation was ensured by conducting weekly supervision with Health Educators, monthly team meetings, and annual re-trainings. Additionally, there were 25 Adverse Events that were managed and systematically reported; all were to protect participants from harm and none were related to study participation. Most adverse events were related to self-reported symptoms of depression, self-harm (cutting), and suicidality.

Results

Effectiveness

Effectiveness, the next phase, is dependent on proper implementation. Effectiveness is the impact of an intervention. The key question is "Are the planned outcomes of the intervention achieved?" This was accomplished by: (1) the development of baseline and follow-up assessments; and (2) the creation and maintenance of an elaborate tracking system. Primary findings from the current study will be published in a forthcoming manuscript. Preliminary results showed that participants who were older and had unemployed mothers demonstrated greater and more frequent substance use at baseline. Additionally, results show that at baseline there was a statistically significant protective relationship between Native Reliance and substance use. Specifically, on average, for every unit increase in Native Reliance, lifetime alcohol use at baseline decreased .8 units, and lifetime marijuana use decreased .78 units. Additionally, results showed that after controlling for baseline use, participants assigned to the active condition (BA+PFR+MI) reported greater reductions ($\beta = -.11$, $p < .01$) in marijuana use at 3 months post baseline than the control condition (BA+PFR). At the 12-month follow-up assessment, participants (n = 89) were asked to complete a Participant Satisfaction Survey; the results were overwhelmingly positive with 100% sating that they "liked the program;" 91% reporting that they found the program "helpful," of which 36% found it "very helpful;" 97% reporting that the Health Educators were "always accepting;" and 92% liked the materials used. These results were shared with stakeholders after the conclusion of the project.

Maintenance

Maintenance in the RE-AIM framework is the extent to which a program becomes institutionalized. The key questions are "Is the intervention sustainable over the long term?" and "Does the program produce lasting effects?" This was accomplished by: (1) biannual CAB meetings and (2) annual trainings of Health Educators. As the project progressed and evolved, several adaptations were necessary. Since many schools were small in terms of enrollment, saturation was often reached quickly, so additional schools were added and the project was extended to another tribe. The additional tribe was represented by a member of the CAB who had heritage, affiliation, and cultural knowledge from both tribes. This member provided input into materials and processes that were used for the intervention. At the request of the schools and CAB, inclusion criteria were expanded to include 12th graders; they were originally excluded to ensure higher long-term response rates at 12-months. To address issues of trust and confidentiality, a brief "getting to know you session" for the Health Educator and participant was added and white noise machines were purchased. Additionally, as time and drug trends changed, the assessments were edited accordingly. Maintenance is, of course, dependent on funding; however, 405 participants were reached across 6 schools in 2 counties and 15 Health Educators were trained, many of whom report continuing to use the MI skills acquired during SACRED Connections.

Discussion, challenges, limitations, and conclusions

Thus far, the first aim of the study has been accomplished: The three intervention conditions (BA +PFR, BA+PFR+MI, and BA+PFR+MI+BOOST) were implemented as intended and compared. Aims 2 (To evaluate the impact of a 6-months-post-intervention booster session on substance use and substance-related negative consequences), 3 (To examine putative mechanisms of change (i.e., mediators) associated with response to our motivational interviewing intervention), and (4) (To explore gender and Native American cultural variables as moderators of intervention response), have not yet been explored.

Overall impact, while not formally included as a dimension of the RE-AIM framework, is proposed as part of the framework as being conceptually helpful to discuss implications and future implementation on a larger scale. Overall impact is defined as the public health impact of the program. This project achieved several successes and great impact, including: the forming of a successful university/NA partnership that resulted in several project goals being attained; the development of a culturally tailored and scientifically sound protocol and materials; engagement of tribal and community leaders and public schools with predominantly NA students; and a brief, substance use intervention offered to 405 NA youth who may not otherwise have received services.

The findings that there was a statistically significant protective relationship between Native Reliance and substance use is an important scientific advance and should be considered in future studies with Native Americans. In their systematic review of risk and protective factors with American Indian and Alaska Native youth, Burnette and Figley (2016) found that there was a lack of consensus in the literature; while they attributed this to difficulties in measurement, they concluded that this was a "severe limitation."

Challenges

University and community partnerships require more time and training than traditional research projects. Following the recommendation of the CAB, NA community members with expertise in substance use counseling reviewed the intervention materials and participated in mock sessions.

Consistent with cultural traditions, they often brought additional counselors. The challenge to the project was in adjusting the timeline to accommodate these additions and resulting changes as well as creatively reallocating and finding additional resources to cover efforts by all involved. A particular challenge was meeting the cultural expectation of shared food, which is often an expense minimally covered by federal grants or not allowed at all. Future funding opportunities for NA research can take this into consideration and allow for such expenses to be built into the budget.

Limitations

While the Native Reliance measure addressed some of the documented measurement limitations, there were other limitations that must be acknowledged. Participant recruitment was limited to public high schools with large enrollments of NA youth from two rural counties in the Midwest, and from predominantly three tribal nations. NA are a heterogeneous group; we do not know how generalizable our findings are to NA youth living in more urban settings or on reservations, in other geographic areas, or with different tribal affiliations. Our MI intervention was limited to individual sessions with participants, and did not involve contact with parents, family, or peers, all of whom are powerful social influences on adolescent substance use. Relatedly, our primary data source was limited to participating adolescents; we did not collect data from parents, teachers, or peers. Additional data sources may help future studies better understand the depth and breadth of MI effects, as well as factors that may moderate effectiveness. Finally, our intervention sessions were limited to school settings and school hours. Among students with substance use problems, tardiness, repeated absences, and truancy are common, complicating the attempts to meet at school. Future studies should consider adding a home-based, non-school-based, and/or after-hours option for MI implementation among students who miss sessions because they miss school.

Conclusions

As supported by the literature (Getty, 2010; Liddell & Burnette, 2017; Marsiglia & Booth, 2015), the partnership between the researchers and the tribal community was critical to the success of this project and resulted in effective cultural tailoring. The partnership with the tribal community ensured that NA cultural values were integrated into implementation and not simply acknowledged (Burnette & Figley, 2016; Whitbeck, 2006; Whitbeck et al., 2012), which facilitated tribal community ownership (Whitbeck, 2006). D&I science, specifically the RE-AIM model, provided a framework that guided the adaptation of the evidence-based practice, Motivational Interviewing, for implementation allowing for adaptations while still holding to the integrity of the evidence-based practice and supporting "long standing partnerships beyond the term of the research" (Whitbeck, 2006).

Results demonstrated that: (1) a culturally responsive MI-based brief intervention may be effective in reducing substance use among NA youth with statistically significant reductions in marijuana use at 3 months; (2) Native Reliance theory is an appropriate framework and protective factor; and (3) an intentional, well-planned, and flexible university-tribal partnership utilizing CBPR methods and a D&I model allowed effective implementation and engagement with a hard to reach underserved community.

Acknowledgments

The authors would like to acknowledge NIDA (1R01DA029779-01A1; MPI's: Wagner & Lowe), NIMHD (1U54MD012393-01; PI: Wagner), and the Training Institute on Dissemination and Implementation Research in Health (NCI & US Department of Veteran's Affairs) funding, support, and training of this research project. They also extend gratitude to the staff of FIU-CBRI (including Robbert Langwerden for his assistance with the preparation of this manuscript), FSU-INRHE, and most importantly, to their tribal partners, elders, Community Advisory Board members, schools, participants, and project staff.

Disclosure statement

No potential conflict of interest was reported by the authors.

Funding

This work was supported by the National Institute on Drug Abuse [1R01DA029779-01A1]; National Institute on Minority Health and Health Disparities [U54MD012393-01].

References

Annis, H. M., & Graham, J. M. (1988). *Situational Confidence Questionnaire (SCQ-39): User's guide.* Addiction Research Foundation.

Arkowitz, H., Miller, W. R., & Rollnick, S. (Eds.). (2015). *Motivational interviewing in the treatment of psychological problems* (2nd ed.). Guilford Press.

Bachman, J. G., Wallace, J. M., Jr., O'Malley, P. M., Johnston, L. D., Kurth, C. L., & Neighbors, H. W. (1991). Racial/ethnic differences in smoking, drinking, and illicit drug use among American high school seniors, 1976–89. *American Journal of Public Health, 81*(3), 372–377. https://doi.org/10.2105/AJPH.81.3.372

Baciu, A., Negussie, Y., & Geller, A. (Eds.). (2017). *Communities in action: Pathways to health equity: The state of health disparities in the United States.* National Academies Press. Retrieved from https://www.ncbi.nlm.nih.gov/books/NBK425844/

Batliner, T., Fehringer, K. A., Tiwari, T., Henderson, W. G., Wilson, A., Brega, A. G., & Albino, J. (2014). Motivational interviewing with American Indian mothers to prevent early childhood caries: Study design and methodology of a randomized control trial. *Trials, 15*(1), 125. https://doi.org/10.1186/1745-6215-15-125

Beauvais, P. (1996). Trends in drug use among American Indian students and dropouts, 1975 to 1994. *American Journal of Public Health, 86*(11), 1594–1598. https://doi.org/10.2105/AJPH.86.11.1594

Borsari, B., & Carey, K. B. (2000). Effects of a brief motivational intervention with college student drinkers. *Journal of Consulting and Clinical Psychology, 68*(4), 728–733. https://doi.org/10.1037/0022-006X.68.4.728

Brave Heart, M. Y. H. (1999). Oyate Ptayela: Rebuilding the Lakota Nation through addressing historical trauma among Lakota parents. *Journal Of Human Behavior In The Social Environment, 2*(1–2), 109–126. https://doi.org/10.1300/J137v02n01_08

Brave Heart, M. Y. H., & DeBruyn, L. M. (1998). The American Indian holocaust: Healing historical unresolved grief. *American Indian and Alaska Native Mental Health Research, 8*(2), 56–78. doi:10.5820/aian.0802.1998.60

Burnette, C. E., & Figley, C. R. (2016). Risk and protective factors related to the wellness of American Indian and Alaska Native youth: A systematic review. *International Public Health Journal, 8*(2), 58–75.

Center for Behavioral Health Statistics and Quality (CBHSQ), SAMHSA & US HHS. (2011). *Results from the 2010 National survey on drug use and health: Summary of national findings*, 1–69. Retrieved from http://archive.samhsa.gov/data/%20NSDUH/2k10nsduh/2k10results.htm

Centers for Disease Control and Prevention (CDC). (2014). *American Indian & Alaska Native populations: Ten leading causes of death.* Retrieved from https://www.cdc.gov/%20minorityhealth/%20populations/REMP/aian.html

Cummings Graduate Institute, CORE: Cummings Online Resources. (2015–2019). *Elements of the RE-AIM Framework Phoenix [Image].* Retrieved from https://azhin.org/cummings/re-aim

D'Amico, E. J., Miles, J. N. V., Stern, S. A., & Meredith, L. S. (2008). Brief motivational interviewing for teens at risk of substance use consequences: A randomized pilot study in a primary care clinic. *Journal of Substance Abuse Treatment, 35*(1), 53–61. https://doi.org/10.1016/j.jsat.2007.08.008

D'Amico, E. J., Parast, L., Shadel, W. G., Meredith, L. S., Seelam, R., & Stein, B. D. (2018). Brief motivational interviewing intervention to reduce alcohol and marijuana use for at-risk adolescents in primary care. *Journal of Consulting and Clinical Psychology, 86*(9), 775. https://doi.org/10.1037/ccp0000332

Daeppen, J. B., Bertholeta, N., Gaumea, J., Fortinia, C., Faouzia, M., & Gmelabc, G. (2011). Efficacy of brief motivational intervention in reducing binge drinking in young men: A randomized controlled trial. *Drug and Alcohol Dependence, 113*(1), 69–75. https://doi.org/10.1016/j.drugalcdep.2010.07.009

Dickerson, D., Baldwin, J. A., Belcourt, A., Belone, L., Gittelsohn, J., Keawe'aimoku Kaholokula, J., Lowe, J., Patten, C. A., & Wallerstein, N. (2018). Encompassing cultural contexts within scientific research methodologies in the development of health promotion interventions. *Prevention Science, 21*(1), 1–10. https://doi.org/10.1007/s11121-018-0926-1

Dickerson, D. L., Brown, R. A., Johnson, C. L., Schweigman, K., & D'Amico, E. J. (2016). Integrating motivational interviewing and traditional practices to address alcohol and drug use among Urban American Indian/Alaska Native Youth. *Journal of Substance Abuse Treatment, 65*, 26–35. https://doi.org/10.1016/j.jsat.2015.06.023

Getty, G. A. (2010). The journey between western and Indigenous research paradigms. *Journal of Transcultural Nursing, 21*(1), 5–14. https://doi.org/10.1177/1043659609349062

Gfellner, B. M., & Hundleby, J. D. (1995). Patterns of drug use among Native and White adolescents: 1990–1993. *Canadian Journal of Public Health*, 86(2), 95–97. www.jstor.org/stable/41991256

Gilder, D. A., Luna, J. A., Calac, D., Moore, R. S., Monti, P. M., & Ehlers, C. L. (2011). Acceptability of the use of motivational interviewing to reduce underage drinking in a Native American Community. *Substance Use & Misuse*, 46(6), 836–842. https://doi.org/10.3109/10826084.2010.541963

Gutierres, S. E., Russo, N. F., & Urbanski, L. (1994). Sociocultural and psychological factors in American Indian drug use: Implications for treatment. *International Journal of the Addictions*, 29(14), 1761–1786. https://doi.org/10.3109/10826089409128256

Guttmannova, K., Wheeler, M. J., Hill, K. G., Evans-Campbell, T. A., Hartigan, L. A., Jones, T. M., Hawkins, J. D., & Catalano, R. F. (2017). Assessment of risk and protection in Native American youth: Steps toward conducting culturally relevant, sustainable, prevention in Indian country. *Journal of Community Psychology*, 45(3), 346. https://doi.org/10.1002/jcop.21852

Harden, S. M., Smith, M. L., Ory, M. G., Smith-Ray, R. L., Estabrooks, P. A., & Glasgow, R. E. (2018). RE-AIM in clinical, community, and corporate Settings: Perspectives, strategies, and recommendations to enhance public health impact. *Frontiers in Public Health*, 6(71). https://doi.org/10.3389/fpubh.2018.00071

Israel, B., Schulz, A., Parker, E., Becker, A., Allen, A., & Guzman, J. R. (2003). Critical issues in developing and following community based participatory principles. In M. Minkler & N. Wallerstein (Eds.), *Community-based participatory research for health* (pp. 53–76). Jossey-Bass/Wiley.

Jessica Liddell & Catherine E. Burnette (2017). Culturally-Informed Interventions for Substance Abuse Among Indigenous Youth in the United States: A Review, Journal of Evidence-Informed Social Work,14:5, 329-359, DOI: 10.1080/23761407.2017.1335631

Kessler, R. C., Wittchen, H. U., Abelson, J. M., McGonagle, K., Schwarz, N., Kendler, K., Knauper, B., & Zhao, S. (1998). Methodological studies of the Composite International Diagnostic Interview (CIDI) in the U.S. National Comorbidity Survey (NCS). *International Journal of Methods in Psychiatric Research*, 7(1), 33–55. https://doi.org/10.1002/mpr.33

Larimer, M. E., Turner, A. P., Anderson, B. K., Fader, J. S., Kilmer, J. R., Palmer, R. S., & Cronce, J. M. (2001). Evaluating a brief alcohol intervention with fraternities. *Journal of Studies on Alcohol*, 62(3), 370–380. https://doi.org/10.15288/jsa.2001.62.370

Lowe, J. (2002). Cherokee Self-Reliance. *Journal of Transcultural Nursing*, 13(4), 287–295. https://doi.org/10.1177/104365902236703

Lowe, J., Liang, H., & Henson, J. (2016). Preventing substance use among Native American early adolescents. *Journal of Community Psychology*, 44(8), 997–1010. https://doi.org/10.1002/jcop.21823

Lowe, J., Wagner, E., Hospital, M. M., Morris, S. L., Thompson, M., Sawant, M., Kelley, M., & Millender, M. (2019). Utility of the native-reliance theoretical framework, model, and questionnaire. *Journal of Cultural Diversity*, 26(2), 61–68.

Marsiglia, F. F., & Booth, J. M. (2015). Cultural adaptation of interventions in real practice settings. *Research on Social Work Practice*, 25(4), 423–432. https://doi.org/10.1177/1049731514535989

Martin, G., Copeland, J., & Swift, W. (2005). The adolescent cannabis check-up: Feasibility of a brief intervention for young cannabis users. *Journal of Substance Abuse Treatment*, 29(3), 207–213. https://doi.org/10.1016/j.jsat.2005.06.005

McCambridge, J., & Strang, J. (2004). The efficacy of a single-session motivational interviewing in reducing drug consumption and perceptions of drug-related risk and harm among young people: Results from a multi-site cluster randomized trial. *Addiction*, 99(1), 39–52. https://doi.org/10.1111/j.1360-0443.2004.00564.x

McCambridge, J., & Strang, J. (2005). Deterioration over time in effect of Motivational Interviewing in reducing drug consumption and related risk among young people. *Addiction*, 100(4), 470–478. https://doi.org/10.1111/j.1360-0443.2005.01013.x

McLennan, J. (1990). Clients' perceptions of counsellors: A brief measure for use in counselling research, evaluation, and training. *Australian Psychologist*, 25(2), 133–146. https://doi.org/10.1080/00050069008260007

Miller, W, &: *Motivational interviewing: preparing people for change*. 2002, New York: Guildford Press, 2

Miller, W.R., & Rollnick, S. Motivational Interviewing: *Preparing people to change addictive behavior*. New York: Guilford Press, 1991.

Monti, P. M., Colby, S. M., Barnett, N. P., Spirito, A., Rohsenow, D. J., Myers, M., Woolard, R., & Lewander, W. (1999). Brief intervention for harm reduction with alcohol-positive older adolescents in a hospital emergency department. *Journal of Consulting and Clinical Psychology*, 67(6), 989–994. https://doi.org/10.1037/0022-006X.67.6.989

Morris, S. L., & Wagner, E. F. (2007). Adolescent substance use: Developmental considerations. (Monograph Series #1). Florida Certification Board/Southern Coast Addiction Technology Transfer Center Network.

Newton, A. S., Mushquash, S., Krank, M., Wild, C., Dyson, M. P., Hartling, L., & Stewart, S. H. (2018). When and how do brief alcohol interventions in primary care reduce alcohol use and alcohol-related consequences among adolescents? *The Journal of Pediatrics*, 197, 221–232. https://doi.org/10.1016/j.jpeds.2018.02.002

Pearlin, L. I., Aneshensel, C. S., & LeBlanc, A. J. (1997). The forms and mechanisms of stress proliferation: The case of AIDS caregivers. *Journal of Health and Social Behavior*, 38(3), 223–236. re-aim.org, 2017. Retrieved from http://www.re-aim.org/

Roberts, L. J., Neal, D. J., Kivlahan, D. R., Baer, J. S., & Marlatt, G. A. (2000). Individual drinking changes following a brief intervention among college students: Clinical significance in an indicated preventive context. *Journal of Consulting and Clinical Psychology*, 68(3), 500–505. https://doi.org/10.1037/0022-006X.68.3.500

Rollnick, S., Mason, P., & Butler, C. (1999). *Health behavior change: A guide for practitioners.* Elsevier Health Sciences.

Schinke, S. P., Tepavac, L., & Cole, K. C. (2000). Preventing substance use among Native American youth: Three-year results. *Addictive Behaviors, 25*(3), 387–397. https://doi.org/10.1016/S0306-4603(99)00071-4

Snijder, M., Stapinski, L., Lees, B., Newton, N., Champion, K., Chapman, C., Ward, J., & Teesson, M. (2018). Substance use prevention programs for Indigenous adolescents in the USA, Canada, Australia and New Zealand: Protocol for a systematic review. *Journal of Medical Internet Research, 7*(2). doi:10.2196/resprot.9012

Sobell, L. C., & Sobell, M. B. (Eds.). (1992). *Timeline Followback: A technique for assessing self-reported alcohol consumption.* Humana Press.

Sobell, L. C., & Sobell, M. B. (1996). *Timeline Followback users' manual for alcohol use.* Addiction Research Foundation.

Sobell, L. C., Sobell, M. B., & Ward, E. (Eds.). (1980). *Evaluating alcohol and drug abuse treatment effectiveness: Recent advances.* Elsevier.

Stein, L. A. R., Colby, S. M., Barnett, N. P., Monti, P. M., Golembeske, C., & Lebeau-Craven, R. (2006). Effects of motivational interviewing for incarcerated adolescents on driving under the influence after release. *American Journal of Addictions, 15*(S1), 50–57. https://doi.org/10.1080/10550490601003680

Substance Abuse and Mental Health Services Administration (SAMHSA). (2004). *Risk and protective factors for substance use among American Indian or Alaska Native youths* (The NSDUH Report, September 24).

Substance Abuse and Mental Health Services Administration (SAMHSA). (2008). *Results from the 2007 national survey on drug use and health: National findings.*

Substance Abuse and Mental Health Services Administration (SAMHSA). (2015). *2012 National Survey on Drug Use and Health (NSDUH).* Retrieved from https://www.samhsa.gov/data/sites/default/files/NSDUH-DetTabs-2015/NSDUH-DetTabs-2015/NSDUH-DetTabs-2015.pdf

Substance Abuse and Mental Health Services Administration (SAMHSA). (2019). *Behavioral health barometer: United States, Volume 5: Indicators as measured through the 2017 National Survey on Drug Use and Health and the National Survey of Substance Abuse Treatment Services.* HHS Publication No. SMA–19–Baro-17-US.

Tarter, R. (1990). *The drug use screening inventory-revised.* Gordian Group.

Urban Indian Health Institute. (2014b). *Supporting sobriety among American Indians and Alaska Natives: A literature review.*

Urban Indian Health Institute (UIHI). (2011). *Community health profile: National aggregate of Urban Indian Health Organization Service Areas.* Retrieved from http://www.uihi.org/wp-content/uploads/2011/12/Combined-UIHO-CHP_Final.pdf

Urban Indian Health Institute (UIHI). (2014a). *Facts sheet.* Retrieved from http://www.uihi.org/wp-content/uploads/2012/11/Fact-sheet_NHIS_Healthcare-access-and-use.pdf

U.S. Department of Health and Human Services, Office of Minority Health (2019). The National CLAS Standards: A blueprint for action. Retrieved from https://www.thinkculturalhealth.hhs.gov/assets/pdfs/EnhancedCLASStandardsBlueprint.pdf

Venner, K. L., Feldstein, S. W., & Tafoya, N. (2017). Helping clients feel welcome: Principles of adapting treatment cross-culturally. *Alcoholism Treatment Quarterly, 25*(4), 11–30. https://doi.org/10.1300/J020v25n04_02

Vinson, C. A., Stamatakis, K. A., & Kerner, J. F. (2017). Dissemination and implementation research in community and public health settings. In R. C. G. Brownson & E. Proctor (Eds.), *Dissemination and implementation research in health* (pp. 359–383). Oxford Press.

Wagner, E. F., Lowe, J., & Baldwin, J. A. (in press). Prevention of substance use disorders in Native Americans. To appear in In C. A. Downey & E. C. Chang (Eds.), *Historical context and cultural competence in substance use disorder* (Chapter 14). American Psychological Association.

Walker, D. D., Roffman, R. A., Stephens, R. S., Berghuis, J. A., & Kim, W. (2006). Motivational enhancement therapy for adolescent marijuana users: A preliminary randomized controlled trial. *Journal of Consulting and Clinical Psychology, 74*(3), 628–632. https://doi.org/10.1037/0022-006X.74.3.628

Wallerstein, N., & Duran, B. (2003). The conceptual, historical and practice roots of community based participatory research and related participatory traditions. In M. Minkler & N. Wallerstein (Eds.), *Community-based participatory research for health* (pp. 27–52). Jossey-Bass/Wiley.

Wallerstein, N., & Duran, B. (2010). Community-based participatory research contributions to intervention research: The intersection of science and practice to improve health equity. *American Journal of Public Health, 100*(S1), 40–46. https://doi.org/10.2105/AJPH.2009.184036

Whitbeck, L. B. (2006). Some guiding assumptions and a theoretical model for developing culturally specific preventions with Native American people. *Journal of Community Psychology, 34*(2), 183–192. https://doi.org/10.1002/jcop.20094

Whitbeck, L. B., Walls, M. L., & Welch, M. L. (2012). Substance abuse prevention in American Indian and Alaska Native communities. *The American Journal of Drug and Alcohol Abuse, 38*(5), 428–435. https://doi.org/10.3109/00952990.2012.695416

Winters, K. C. (1991). *The personal experience screening questionnaire.* Western Psychological Services.

From myPlan to ourCircle: Adapting a web-based safety planning intervention for Native American women exposed to intimate partner violence

Meredith E. Bagwell-Gray, Em Loerzel, Gail Dana Sacco, Jill Messing ⓘ,
Nancy Glass, Bushra Sabri ⓘ, Brittany Wenniserí:iostha Jock, Joyell Arscott,
Teresa Brockie, and Jacquelyn Campbell

ABSTRACT

This paper describes the adaptation of a web-based safety planning intervention for Native American women exposed to intimate partner violence (IPV). We conducted interviews with Native American women exposed to intimate partner violence (*n* = 40) and practitioners who work with Native American survivors (*n* = 41) to gain an understanding of culturally specific risk and protective factors for IPV. Participants were from three regions of the U.S. – the Northeast, Southeast, and Southwest – from a mixture of rural (reservation and non-reservation) and urban settings. These data were then used to inform culturally responsive adaptation of a web-based safety app, called myPlan (renamed ourCircle) by infusing it with culturally specific safety priorities and safety strategies. This research has implications for the Grand Challenges for Social Work, specifically the Challenges to End Family Violence, Harness Technology for Social Good, and Achieve Equal Opportunity and Justice.

Native American women experience higher rates of intimate partner violence (IPV) in comparison to women from other racial and ethnic backgrounds (Black et al., 2011). It is estimated that 37.5% of Native American women experience IPV within their lifetime, as compared to 29.1% for Black women, 24.8% for White women, and 15% for Asian women (Black et al., 2011; Finfgeld-Connett, 2015). Disparate rates of IPV are best understood within the context of historical oppression, wherein past and present trauma experienced by groups of people with a shared identity have cumulative and intergenerational impacts on their health outcomes (Burnette, 2015; Evans-Campbell, 2008). Over time, violence impacts future generations of family and community in ways broader than the direct impact of violence, with one generation experiencing violence and passing it to the next, which can normalize violence in the community (Burnette, 2015). Ultimately, the impact of historical oppression and its symptoms, such as PTSD, suicidality, and aggressive behavior, and its downstream effects, such as child abuse, substance use, and community breakdown, can be exacerbated by the experience of present-day trauma and IPV (Brockie et al., 2015). This theoretical frame expands the notion of individual trauma (e.g., PTSD) on communities and populations by examining the social impact of intergenerational trauma with proximal and contemporary oppressive events, while acknowledging the resilience of the affected communities (Duran, 2006; Evans-Campbell, 2008).

Historical oppression and intergenerational trauma are compatible with a health disparities framework of understanding violence again Native women, which locates immediate risk factors in the distal social environment in addition to the proximal social environment. While biology and life experiences have a role in someone's susceptibility to negative health outcomes (Cordero et al., 2012; Smith et al., 2011), individual and interpersonal attributes are inadequate at explaining health disparities (Gehlert et al., 2008).

During colonization, many tribes were forcibly removed far from their lands to reservations west of the Mississippi (Huyser et al., 2014). These reservations, often located in remote areas that are economically and socially isolated (Mathers, 2012), created communities with limited job opportunities, high rates of unemployment (Huyser et al., 2014; Mathers, 2012), and a high rate of poverty compared to average families in the U.S. (39.1% versus 29.0%; Huyser et al., 2014). It was often the goal of settlers to assimilate or eradicate the Indigenous peoples and their culture to gain control of resources (Le May, 2018). Colonizers created laws, social norms, and policies that promoted violence against Indigenous people including murder (i.e., the scalping of Native Americans by settler bounty hunters in exchange for monetary value), removing the community's men (i.e., discriminatory and regressive criminal and incarceration policies), and forcefully taking Indigenous women as partners to eradicate Native culture (Le May, 2018). The power of Indigenous women in traditional societies threatened colonizing patriarchal systems; thus, violence against Indigenous women functioned as a tool of colonization (Smith, 2015). Introducing European gender roles into matriarchal or egalitarian-ran tribal communities ensured Native American women's voices were disenfranchised, thereby increasing vulnerability to violence and exploitation (Le May, 2018).

High rates of IPV among Native American women and the historical context of colonizing violence indicate an urgent need for IPV interventions that are culturally tailored for Native American women, particularly those that build upon strengths and protective factors (Yuan et al., 2015). The purpose of this paper is to describe an adaptation of an online safety planning intervention (myPlan) for Native American women. The adaptation process was informed by qualitative research, the goal of which was to better understand culturally specific risk and protective factors to inform culturally responsive safety priorities and safety strategies. The guiding research question was: What are the culturally specific risk and protective factors for lethal and near-lethal violence for Native American women?

Background intervention: why the myPlan web app?

The myPlan web app (www.myplanapp.org) is a secure, interactive, and personalized app that has been developed and tested with diverse women-identified survivors of partner violence to support decisions to increase safety and reduce barriers to multiple services including advocacy hotlines and programs, legal, housing and health (Glass et al., 2017; Koziol-McLain et al., 2018). myPlan users assess their level of danger using the Danger Assessment, a validated risk assessment for intimate partner homicide (Campbell et al., 2003), and are provided with information on their level of danger. In the interactive decision aid, the user weighs their priorities (e.g., safety for themselves, love for their partner, privacy) and receives immediate feedback on the things that are most important to them. The app then uses this user input to formulate a personally tailored safety plan with links to resources and services.

In a longitudinal randomized control trial (RCT) using the internet-based version of myPlan (previously known as IRIS), diverse abused women (40% racial/ethnic minorities and 10% sexual minorities) who used myPlan reported reductions in decisional conflict (e.g., the user feels more certain in decisions, more clear on priorities, and more supported) and an increased use of helpful safety behaviors, such as talking or texting with IPV service providers when compared to women in the control group (e.g., information and a standard safety plan; Eden et al., 2015; Glass et al., 2017). Additionally, women in the intervention group were more likely to decide to end the abusive relationship during the study period (12 months), report that the safety strategies they used were helpful, and experience less psychological abuse and sexual violence compared to the control group (Glass et al., 2017).

The growing support for myPlan as an evidence-based intervention motivates our current work to adapt it for Native American women experiencing IPV. This work is particularly relevant because internet- and mobile-based technologies can improve health and mental health outcomes for women in rural areas who face barriers to accessing resources (Braun et al., 2014). myPlan has been adapted and tested in New Zealand among both non-Maori and Indigenous Maori women (iSafe), Australia (iDecide), Canada (iCan), Kenya (myPlan Kenya). It is currently being adapted for teens ages 15 to 17 and women in Kyrgyzstan. The adaptation tested among Indigenous Maori women has been shown to be effective in reducing repeat violence (Koziol-McLain et al., 2018). By engaging in collaboration with community members and stakeholders during cultural adaptation, programming can be tailored to include cultural norms and values, therefore creating a targeted and impactful response to community issues (Marsiglia & Booth, 2014; Okamoto et al., 2013). Not only does this deconstruct the typical Western research hierarchy but it also creates a space for community to have self-autonomy and voice in the research process (Okamoto et al., 2013).

Methods

The purpose of this sequential, mixed methods study was to adapt and test the myPlan intervention for Native American women. This article focuses on findings from the Phase 1 qualitative data that informed the adaptation. IRB approvals were obtained from the two universities collaborating on the project. In addition, the research was approved through the Office of American Indian Projects, gatekeepers to vet university-community collaborative research projects among Native American populations. We also obtained requisite tribal approvals for data collected on tribal lands.

Setting and sample

Phase 1 was conducted in the northeastern, southeastern, and southwestern United States. The primary investigator engaged informal and formal networks to identify and recruit research team members who, based on their experience and interest in conducting community-engaged research with Native American communities, could facilitate building relationships with tribal partners. Three research team members, one in each region, were primarily responsible for recruitment, data collection, and analysis. Two are non-Indigenous white women and one is a Native American woman; all three, who have doctoral degrees, serve as faculty at different academic institutions in the fields of public health or social work. The team member working in the Southeast has been joined in collaborative partnerships with the tribal communities for over a decade. In the Northeast, an Indigenous team member from that area, who has long standing relationships and research experience there and in other Native communities, developed research partnership agreements with tribes.

Based on these relationships, our team collaborated with five tribes in the Northeast, two tribes in the Southeast, and two partner organizations in the Southwest. Advocates and practitioners assisted in disseminating information about the study, actively recruited participants and arranged interviews. Participants included advocates and providers (n = 41) with two or more years of experience serving Native American survivors and Native American women, ages 18 to 64, who self-reported IPV in the past year (n = 42; see Table 1).

Table 1. Participants by region in the Northeast, Southeast and Southwest U.S.

Region	Survivor Interviews	Provider Interview Format		Total
		Focus Groups	Interviews	
Northeast	20	12	0	32
Southeast	9	4	3	16
Southwest	13	17	5	35
Total	42	33	8	83

In the Northeast, participants were rural and reservation based, often having lived in other Native and non-Native communities, both rural and urban. In the Southeast, one tribe was situated in a primarily rural setting and the other was a mixture of rural and urban. In the Southwest, one partner organization was in an urban setting and one was in a rural area bordering a reservation.

Data collection

Data collection, in the form of individual interviews and focus groups, occurred between July 2016 and June 2017. All interviews and focus groups were semi-structured. The interview guide, which covered risk factors, strengths and protective factors, was developed by one of the investigators based on her expertise on IPV and related health inequities (see Table 2). Interview and focus group sessions lasted approximately 60 to 90 minutes, except for one focus group, conducted in two sessions, which lasted approximately 3 hours long. Sessions were audio-recorded and transcribed. Participants received a financial stipend for participation. Survivors received 35 USD and practitioners received 40 USD; this difference accounts for practitioners' additional role in disseminating study information to help recruit survivors.

Table 2. Example interview questions from the interview guide.

Risk Factors

Prompt: *Some women are in situations where they fear being severely attacked, or even killed by their husband/partner because of things he says or does. In this interview, I'd like your help in identifying what some of these risk factors or warning signs might be, so other Native American women can understand the risks they might face. "Risk factors" is another way of saying red-flags or warning signs.*

- Are there any red flags or warning signs in your relationship that make you think that things may be getting more dangerous, like he might try to seriously hurt or even kill you?
- Which risk factors did you find to be the most important for you [or in your community]?
- Why do you believe these risk factors to be the most important?

Safety Strategies

- What are some of the ways that you kept yourself safe?
- Did these strategies help/make you safer? Why or why not?
- Are there people in your life that help you stay safer?
- How do you think that your enculturation (i.e., extent to which you are connected with Native ways of life) affects your safety? Why do you say that?

Unique Strengths

- What do you believe are some of your characteristics or beliefs that have helped you as a survivor? What makes you think that? How did you use these strengths to your advantage? Tell me about that.

Data analysis

We used Dedoose to store and manage data. The three research team members who collected the data reviewed audio-recordings and transcripts and, using thematic analysis (Braun & Clarke, 2006), identified risk and protective factors for IPV, focusing on culturally specific contexts of Native American women's lives. With these perspectives, the researchers met with a full team, comprised of both Native American and non-Native American researchers from the fields of nursing, social work, and public health, for a 3-day, in-person working retreat. During this retreat, research team members reviewed emerging themes to develop myPlan adaptations. These results highlight risk and protective factors in participants' words with corresponding changes in the adaptation denoted by textboxes.

Results

Risk factor: interrupted connections with native identify and culture

Some abusive partners prevented (or tried to prevent) women from connecting with their Native identity or culture. When abusive partners were non-Native, this happened by not allowing women to speak their Native language or practice their tribal spirituality:

> I always spoke [our Native language] to [my daughter], ever since she was born. [My abusive partner] doesn't like that. If I said [a word in Native language] to her, he's like, "It's water. Just tell her it's water." ... He didn't want me teachin' her that stuff. Language is very important to me. That's where I get a lot of pride from.

This participants' quotation demonstrates great resiliency and strength in her pride for her language. Even though her partner attempted to keep her from connecting, she persisted, demonstrating resilience.

In other examples, some abusive partners who were Native American expressed ethnic bias toward their partners if they were members of different tribes or nations:

> He would tell me, "You're not cooking it right," ... He'd throw it across the room ... I'd go up there during ceremonies ... and nobody would eat ... cuz I was [name of tribe]. They wanted a [name of another tribe] woman cooking.

In this example, the participant did not have a sense of belonging in the tribal community in which she lived because her heritage was from multiple tribes. This lack of belonging, and the prejudice experienced by her partner and his family, limited her ability to participate in tribal traditions and ceremonies, practices that could serve as protective factors.

Protective factor: honoring native identity and culture

Providers in one focus group contrasted this risk factor with a parallel protective factor. They spoke of healthy relationships in which both partners honor one another's spiritual practices and cultural heritage, even when they differ:

> He really wants his kids to be traditional, know the traditions, practice them. She's not so much on board. They have a good balance … They actually really respect each other … There was a time that the son was having trouble because he kept speaking English and [tribal language] at the same time in his kindergarten. I remember her being a little upset about that, but she still hung in there and said, "It's equally important."

This example demonstrates that a true sign of respect in a relationship among couples necessitates valuing one another's heritage and supporting one another's participation in traditional practices.

Corresponding change

myPlan has a list of attributes found in healthy relationships. In the ourCircle adaptation, we added an attribute of healthy relationships entitled Cultural and Spiritual Responsibility.

ourCircle App: Cultural and Spiritual Responsibility: Both partners honor one another's role in carrying out cultural and spiritual responsibilities.

Risk factor: when leaving the abuse means leaving home

Participants said that for some women, choosing to leave an abusive relationship would mean leaving their homeland: "When you have a strong tie to your community, you haven't left. You live there. Leaving that relationship means you probably have to leave your home." This risk was tied to the fact that women desired to maintain social relationships in large, extended families, including their own families and their partners' families. Caring for families was one of the most important priorities and values, shaping what it meant to be a woman in the community: "You take care of your family. … That's how it's always been with my grandmother and my mother and all of the people – all of the Natives I know. That's always been the top priority."

In these extended social networks, people have a strong interdependence on one another. For example, participants described living with extended family, relying on relatives for childcare, and caregiving for family members, such as aging parents or in-laws. With strong ties to community, the decision to leave an abusive relationship was untenable when doing so would be synonymous with cutting those ties. Thus, mechanisms for establishing safety need to accommodate new approaches that promote healing and account-ability for the abusive partner:

> They wanna do a fix, right? You see [the] westernized way, doing a fix. The fix is they have to leave their perpetrator … Well, that doesn't work so well in Native community. Part of it is trying to get the perpetrator help … We have to start healing those wounds.

Corresponding changes

myPlan has five priorities women often weigh when planning for their safety. In ourCircle, we added a 6th priority: *Connecting to Native Community*. This priority recognizes the value of staying connected to community and helps the user incorporate that value into her safety planning. If a woman ranks this as her top priority, she will see the following prompt:

ourCircle App: Your answers indicate that connecting or restoring connections to your Native community, whether on or off reservation, is what's most important to you. Sometimes experiencing partner violence can interrupt your spiritual and tribal connections. Being in touch with your community and its network of resources can enhance your capacity to cope whether you leave or whether you stay. ourCircle can provide suggestions to help.

There is also an added safety strategy in ourCircle, called *Connecting to the Land/Homeland*:

ourCircle App: One way to connect to your heritage is by visiting the homeland. If that isn't possible, you can learn about your homeland and the history and your people, learn your Indigenous language, and seek out or share traditional food and meals, songs, and stories.

Risk factor: high threshold for red flags

Participants described that another risk factor was not noticing red flags and warning signs until the violence was extremely severe. This risk factor was associated with intergenerational violence and abuse: "It's in my whole family. My mother, my father my aunts, my uncles. One of my aunts was killed by her husband." Some providers described that women accepted the violence because of the normalization of the violence:

> It wasn't seen as a risk as much as something that you bear and something that you walk through and the journey that's going to of course always happen … I've been sitting there with four generations and the advice that's coming from those generations is you just have to put up with it.

As one provider described, the bar is moved for assessing the risk for intimate partner homicide using the danger assessment:

Threats with a weapon, threats to kill, and threats to harm children – that's standard stuff in our community. ... The danger assessment moves. If she's seen her mother, or her grandmother, or her auntie, or her sister have a weapon drawn on her, it's not going to have the same effect.

This providers' comment on the applicability of the danger assessment is sobering given the higher rates of intimate partner homicide among Native American women compared to women of other racial and ethnic identities in the U.S. The myPlan app includes the Danger Assessment (Campbell et al., 2003) and generates a danger assessment score for women to inform their safety planning strategies. This characteristic was kept the same in the ourCircle app, with the anticipation that seeing a risk score, as generated by the Danger Assessment, would disrupt the normalization of extreme levels of violence that are risk indicators of homicide.

Protective factor: social connections with other native women

As a meaningful, relevant protective factor, women described gaining power and protection through their social connections with other Native women:

It's the way we come around each other, especially in a time of need. It's like a blanket, very protective. ... We were somewhere drummin', and this little one says, "How do you know each other?" ... It feels like we've known each other beyond this lifetime, right? That in itself is a connection that I wish for everyone, but is something rare, I think.

Another participant similarly described how women being connected with women acted as a protective factor: "more people are gonna know what's going on with you, know you're in a situation of violence and be there to support [you]." Being connected to community was characterized by matriarchal power structures "where women were more valued and ... respected" and were leaders in the community: "That's something that's tied in with Native culture, is powerful women." Thus, the leadership and connections among Native women demonstrate important answers to the risks posed by intergenerational violence.

Corresponding changes

ourCircle has an additional safety strategy called *Networks* that acknowledges intergenerational violence yet encourages women to build up nonviolent networks in their communities. This strategy reads:

ourCircle App: Trauma and violence within your network are not really tradition, even if it has been passed down from past generations. There are always some people who have a sacred spiritual responsibility in the community who provide direction and guidance toward nonviolence, safety, and peace. Connect with these tribal and relational networks, including extended family and political connections to get to know who your relatives are. Find safe relatives who do not support or contribute to the abuse and strengthen your relationships with them. Standing in the circle is the first step – find a circle to stand in.

Risk factor: challenges balancing native and non-native ways

Participants discussed that a risk factor was balancing Native and non-Native ways of life: "If you're an Indigenous person, there's always that battle of modern and traditional, and it's hard to find people who can fluctuate in both worlds, cuz it literally is two worlds an Indigenous person walks." One of the differences between the two worlds is an emphasis on collectivism:

> When you look at those pieces of merging cultures as a result of this prolonged contact that we have had, we struggle because so often times they're in dire contrast to each other. Where western world is like, you do what you do for yourself and your family, end of story. And here, you do what you do for the tribe first, for the nation first, then the bigger family, which is everyone, and then your family members. You do that to the depth of who you are. Our communities and our spiritual things are all set up – the dances that we do or the ceremonies that we have – are specifically set up to take care of our community.

This excerpt reiterates how important it is that interventions for Native IPV survivors account for collective identity and maintaining community ties. When IPV interventions do not recognize and honor these values, it could further contribute to the struggle that Native women face by forcing them to choose one world (i.e., the western world) over the other. This can result in feeling "confused and lost": "I've felt confused and lost most of my life. I'm [Tribal Affiliation]. That's what I am, so I need to learn about who I am through my culture."

Protective factors: learning cultural ways and practicing traditions

Teaching and learning about cultural ways of living is an important strategy to counteract this risk factor: "If you're connected with traditional values, that decreases your risk of violence … The women who feel connected to their roots, to their identity, to their customs, their risk goes down." Connecting with Native identity or culture was a relevant protective factor that could counteract the challenge of walking in two worlds:

> On the reservation, they would always tell me, 'You're walking in two worlds.' I never really understood what that meant until now. … Now I'm realizing that the important thing is having that identity. Realizing that you can have a dual identity of being traditional and connecting in that way and having that spirituality … Having that balance.

As this participant described, having a strong identity helped find that balance when walking in two worlds. Another strategy for finding balance was through participating in ceremony and traditional spiritual practices:

> Smudging, sweat lodge, drumming, standing as part of that circle, even if you may not be a drummer, but just standing there sometimes helps, reaching out to an elder that may have been there a time or two and has moved beyond it. ... In our community, it's the women that tend to show up for anything and everything ... If there's healing that needs to happen, it's the women that show up to do that ... moving that healing process along.

This quotation demonstrates the linkage between several of the themes: connecting with Native identity or culture, participating in spiritual traditions and practices, and connecting with Native women.

Corresponding changes

Primarily, this cluster of themes demonstrates the impetus for the shift in the name of the intervention from myPlan to ourCircle, as "standing as a part of that circle" is a significant protective factor. The name ourCircle demonstrates the collective nature of empowerment and the connections forged in participating in healing together.

One of the myPlan safety priorities is *Health and Well-being*. Within this priority, ourCircle adds emphasis on spiritual wellbeing by including an option to seek support from a spiritual leader and use spiritual strategies for coping with stress. Furthermore, ourCircle incorporates an additional safety strategy, called *Healing*:

ourCircle App: One important part of healing is finding balance between what is sometimes a tension between Native traditions and non-Native ways of life. This can especially be the case if you have had to leave your home, your family, or your reservation. Connecting with spiritual traditions can be a meaningful aspect of healing. Spiritual traditions provide interconnectedness and balance. Another way of healing is touching the earth and water, connecting with Mother Earth. Touching the earth and water is also a way of connecting with ancestors – when you walk on the earth, you're walking on the bones of your ancestors.

ourCircle also has a related safety strategy called *Indigenous Knowledge*, that is related to the spiritual aspect of participating in ceremony:

ourCircle App: All Native people carry Indigenous knowledge within them. You can awaken to the Indigenous knowledge you carry within you by participating in ceremony. This knowledge can help you choose what is best for you and your family.

Protective factor: resilience in the face of historic and contemporary trauma

The participants described an overwhelming level of resiliency in the face of historic and contemporary trauma. As one participant described: "It's like trauma on top of trauma. And yet we continue to push through this trauma. I think that's one of the things that makes us strong." Another described an antidote to intergenerational trauma through "intergenerational healing":

> Intergenerational healing is about empowering individuals to remember where we came from. [It's a] strengths-based perspective of how culturally rich our people are ... about rejuvenating our cultural practices, our ceremonies, our self-esteem, our sense of self-care. ... You have the ability to address these issues and not pass them to your children.

Discussion

Findings from this study on Native American women's risk and protective factors for IPV fills an important gap in research and practice. As a team, we examined the stories of Indigenous women whose lives had been affected by IPV and then practitioners who work with them in order to adapt an evidence-based intervention (myPlan) for Native American women. We used women's voices to change the name of the app to ourCircle, reflecting the importance of being part of an Indigenous community and the strength that women gain from "standing as part of [the] circle." The edits made to the intervention were discussed extensively among the team at an in-person retreat where we focused on reflecting the resiliencies of Indigenous communities while also accounting for risk arising from colonization and historical oppression.

Our investigation of protective factors informs a strengths-based framework that highlights the resilience that Indigenous women and their communities hold despite historical oppression and intergenerational abuse. This is noteworthy because deficits-based frameworks, which focus on the problems within a community, are more commonly used in research with Indigenous communities (Burnette & Figley, 2016). In order to "decolonize" IPV intervention research and move away from a problem-focused framework, it is important for researchers to rely on the strength, voice, and autonomy of the community while at the same time reject both externalized and internalized messages of oppression that have been instilled by a settler-colonial society (Walters & Simoni, 2009). Thus, frameworks of historical oppression need to include concepts of individual, family and community strengths and resilience. This shift calls for extensive engagement of Native American communities, including community members and tribal leadership (Walters & Simoni, 2009). We gathered the stories and incorporated the voices of Indigenous survivors of violence and practitioners from multiple regions of the U.S., and worked to be thoughtful about the adaptations, yet it is likely that our perspectives as Indigenous and allied researchers affect the interpretation of results and the adaptations to the intervention. One of the key attributes of this team of researchers is that we are a blend of Indigenous and non-Indigenous scholars. Working together means engaging in "cultural exchange," (Palinkas et al., 2009) in which we navigate tensions and build trust with one another. While this has meant challenges, the work led the ourCircle adaptation, a product we are testing in an RCT.

One of the largest challenges in developing a culturally specific intervention is being inclusive toward over 550 federally recognized tribes as well as those that are not federally recognized. We acknowledge the heterogeneity in these Native cultures, yet at the same time, we called upon core commonalities. Evans-Campbell (2008) distinguishes between traumatic events that are shared among many tribes, like boarding schools and relocation to reservations, and tribal-specific traumatic events, like the prohibition of whaling for tribes along the Northwest coast of the U.S. Thus, while it is meaningful that this study is national in scope, it is limited to participating tribes and regions. There is an opportunity for future, community-based research, rooted in the divergent experiences of tribes, to complement these findings.

One limitation to this research is that smartphone and app-based content may not be accessible to women on rural reservation land. Furthermore, this research is limited because the intervention adaptation could be considered a micro-level approach to a macro-level problem, that is, the ourCircle app addresses individuals rather than families, communities, or society. Key elements of prevention and intervention are missed when the environment is not addressed (Whitaker et al., 2008). Coordinated service models that promote empowerment and communication between systems (i.e., criminal justice, shelters, and counseling centers) may compliment individual-level interventions such as ourCricle to provide a safer environment for women who are experiencing IPV (Pennington-Zoellner, 2009). Interventions are also needed with men who use violence to facilitate healing and reduce violence, demonstrating that no single intervention is a panacea; to reduce IPV, intervention requires multiple perspectives.

Despite these limitations, this research lifts the voices of Native American women who have experienced IPV, highlighting their own and their community resiliencies and protective factors. Adapting content to incorporate Indigenous knowledge, healing, networks, connecting to land/homeland, connecting to Native community, and cultural and spiritual responsibility allowed us to make culturally appropriate adaptation of an evidence-based intervention while keeping some core elements of the intervention the same.

Implications for social work and interdisciplinary practice

This research addresses three of the Grand Challenges for Social Work. First, the Grand Challenge "achieving equal opportunity and justice" indicates that social work practitioners have an inherent responsibility and duty to engage with research that meets community needs and empowers them to become autonomous and sovereign. Many social workers, both Native and non-Native service providers, work on tribal lands and in Tribal communities. With many social workers being the "front line" providers to assist victims through the reporting or healing process after IPV, social work plays an important role in advocacy and service provision. With 1% of social workers identifying as Native American (Cross et al., 2010), it is vital that non-Native social workers gain an understanding on Native American tribal jurisdiction and history in order to effectively and ethically provide services to Native American survivors of violence.

The second Grand Challenge that this research addresses, "Harness technology for social good," focuses on the importance of using technology in social work intervention in a manner consistent with the changing nature of technology within society. The ourCircle intervention, following over 10 years of development and testing of the myPlan app, provides a culturally responsive version of a free online intervention for survivors of IPV. IPV is a pervasive social problem, particularly for Native American women, yet women may not understand their danger, feel conflicted about their next steps, and/or not know where to obtain the information and help that they need. ourCircle fills this gap by providing risk assessment, a decision aid, and a tailored safety plan and resources for survivors. ourCircle is not intended to replace social services, but to compliment available interventions and facilitate survivors' use of helpful community resources.

Finally, the Grand Challenge to "End Family Violence" focuses on all forms of violence within the family, including IPV. Given the intergenerational and historical trauma faced by Native American women (Burnette, 2015), the framework of family violence may assist us in understanding the pervasiveness and impact of historical oppression and its symptoms (e.g., child abuse) which can be exacerbated due to IPV (Evans-Campbell, 2008). Yet, the framework of family violence is unable to address the gendered nature of IPV that cannot be overlooked. Nevertheless, this research pulls together three important Grand Challenges through a focus on intervening in IPV with a culturally responsive framework and integration of technology.

Social workers can collaborate with professionals from various disciplines (e.g., social workers, nurses, medical, public health professions) to address safety and health-care needs of Native American survivors of IPV. For instance, primary health-care professionals can play a significant role in early intervention as women typically make multiple visits to health professionals before disclosure (Hegarty, 2018). Health-care professionals can work with professionals from other disciplines to provide needed services to survivors. Integrated care such as availability of specific services for IPV survivors and services addressing trauma in health-care settings may have positive outcomes for Native women. A systematic review of integrated care at Indigenous health-care sites demonstrated positive outcomes such as improved physical and mental health symptoms and reduced substance use (Lewis & Myhra, 2017).

Directions for future research

Then, the next stage of this research is twofold. First, the research team continues to deepen the thematic analysis of phase one data to illuminate risk and protective factors for Indigenous women experiencing intimate partner violence. Second, we are testing the reliability and validity ourCircle and assessing its impact on Indigenous women's empowerment, safety and mental health. Given the context of historical oppression, anti-oppressive research approaches are needed in future research. It is critical that the field of social work and other disciplines examine the disparity of IPV in Native communities using a culturally specific approach rooted in social justice and cultural humility (Gehlert et al., 2008; Matamonasa-Bennett, 2015).

Furthermore, there are important implications for the use of interdisciplinary research teams to address health disparities. Violence is a complex social problem requiring interdisciplinary collaboration to prevent and address negative outcomes (Hegarty, 2018). Diverse perspectives offered by members on the team led to comprehensive and multidimensional analysis of the needs of survivors. Research collaborations may entail having multidisciplinary investigators on the team as well as community stakeholders. All team members offer their unique expertise in the process of research. For instance, researchers can ensure scientific rigor in methods and community partners can facilitate recruitment and help in the interpretation of study findings (Stewart et al., 2007).

In conclusion, scholars and practitioners have a unique opportunity to engage with Native American communities to inform interventions that are evidence-based and culturally responsive. This research process demonstrates how research and practice converge in a way that aligns with our social work values and addresses several social work grand challenges.

Disclosure statement

No potential conflict of interest was reported by the authors.

Funding

This work was supported by the Eunice Kennedy Shriver National Institute of Child Health and Human Development [R01 HD081179-01].

ORCID

Jill Messing ⓘ http://orcid.org/0000-0002-9941-3512
Bushra Sabri ⓘ http://orcid.org/0000-0002-3258-523X

References

Black, M. C., Basile, K. C., Breiding, M. J., Smith, S. G., Walters, M. L., Merrick, M. T., Chen, J., & Stevens, M. R. (2011). *The National Intimate Partner and Sexual Violence Survey (NISVS): 2010 summary report*. National Center for Injury Prevention and Control, Centers for Disease Control and Prevention.

Braun, R., Catalani, C., Wimbush, J., & Israelski, D. (2014). Community health workers and mobile technology: A systematic review of the literature. *PLoS One, 8*(6), e65772. https://doi.org/10.1371/journal.pone.0065772

Braun, V., & Clarke, V. (2006). Using thematic analysis in psychology. *Qualitative Research in Psychology, 3*(2), 77–101. https://doi.org/10.1191/1478088706qp063oa

Brockie, T. B., Dana-Sacco, M., Wallen, G. R., Wilcox, H. C., & Campbell, J. C. (2015). The relationship of adverse childhood experiences to PTSD, depression, poly-drug use and suicide attempt in reservation-based native American adolescents and young adults. *American Journal of Community Psychology, 55*(3–4), 411–421. https://doi.org/10.1007/s10464-015-9721-3

Burnette, C. (2015). Historical oppression and intimate partner violence experienced by indigenous women in the United States: Understanding connections. *Social Service Review, 89*(3), 531–563. https://doi.org/10.1086/683336

Burnette, C. E., & Figley, C. R. (2016). Historical oppression, resilience, and transcendence: Can a holistic framework help explain violence experienced by indigenous people? *Social Work, 62*(1), 37–44. https://doi.org/10.1093/sw/sww065

Campbell, J. C., Webster, D., Koziol-McLain, J., Block, C., Campbell, D., Curry, M. A., Gary, F., Glass, N., McFarlane, J., Sachs, C., & Sharps, P. (2003). Risk factors for femicide in abusive relationships: Results from a multi-site case-control study. *American Journal of Public Health, 93*(7), 1089–1097. https://doi.org/10.2105/AJPH.93.7.1089

Cordero, M. I., Poirier, G. L., Marquez, C., Veenit, V., Fontana, X., Salehi, B., Ansermet, F., & Sandi, C. (2012). Evidence for biological roots in the transgenerational transmission of intimate partner violence. *Translational Psychiatry, 2*(4), e106. https://doi.org/10.1038/tp.2012.32

Cross, S. L., Brown, E. F., Day, P. A., Limb, G. E., Pellebon, D. A., Proctor, E. C., & Weaver, H. N. (2010). Task force on native Americans in social work education. *Council of Social Work Education*.

Duran, E. (2006). *Healing the soul wound: Counselling with American Indians and other native peoples*. (A. E. Ivey & D. W. Sue, Eds.). Teachers College Press.

Eden, K. B., Perrin, N. A., Hanson, G. C., Messing, J. T., Bloom, T. L., Campbell, J. C., Gielen, A. C., Clough, A. S., Barnes-Hoyt, J. S., & Glass, N. E. (2015). Use of online safety decision aid by abused women: Effect on decisional conflict in a randomized controlled trial. *American Journal of Preventive Medicine, 48*(4), 372–383. https://doi.org/10.1016/j. amepre.2014.09.027

Evans-Campbell, T. (2008). Historical Trauma in American Indian/native Alaska communities. *Journal of Interpersonal Violence, 23*(3), 316–338. https://doi.org/10.1177/ 0886260507312290

Finfgeld-Connett, D. (2015). Qualitative systematic review of intimate partner violence among native Americans. *Issues in Mental Health Nursing, 36*(10), 754–760. https://doi. org/10.3109/01612840.2015.1047072

Gehlert, S., Mininger, C., Sohmer, D., & Berg, K. (2008). (Not so) gently down the stream: Choosing targets to ameliorate health disparities. *Health & Social Work, 33*(3), 163–167. https://doi.org/10.1093/hsw/33.3.163

Glass, N. E., Perrin, N. A., Hanson, G. C., Bloom, T. L., Messing, J. T., Clough, A. S., Campbell, J. C., Gielen, A. C., Case, J., & Eden, K. B. (2017). The longitudinal impact of an internet safety decision aid for abused women. *The American Journal of Preventative Medicine, 52*(5), 606–615. https://doi.org/10.1016/j.amepre.2016.12.014

Hegarty, K. (2018). *Strengthening and sustaining the primary care response to family violence: A new model* (Paper #2 of the Safer Families Centre of Research Excellence Discussion Paper Series). http://www.saferfamilies.org.au/discuss

Huyser, K. R., Takei, I., & Sakamoto, A. (2014). Demographic factors associated with poverty among American Indians and Alaska natives. *Race and Social Problems, 6*(2), 120–134. https://doi.org/10.1007/s12552-013-9110-1

Koziol-McLain, J., Vandal, A. C., Wilson, D., Nada-Raja, S., Dobbs, T., McLean, C., & Glass, N. E. (2018). Efficacy of a web-based safety decision aid for women experiencing intimate partner violence: Randomized controlled trial. *Journal of Medical Internet Research, 20*(1), e8.

Le May, G. (2018). Cycles of violence against native women: An analysis of colonialism, historical legislation and the violence against women reauthorization act of 2013. *Portland State University McNair Research Journal, 12*(1), 1-24. *2018.* https://pdxscholar.library.pdx. edu/cgi/viewcontent.cgi?article=1177&context=mcnair

Lewis, M. E., & Myhra, L. L. (2017). Integrated care with indigenous populations: A systematic review of the literature. *American Indian Alaskan Native Mental Health Research, 24*(3), 88110. https://pdfs.semanticscholar.org/ee84/976adbc1ba98e562f3ed847cf1 fad43c25f1.pdf

Marsiglia, F. F., & Booth, J. M. (2014). Cultural adaptation of interventions in real practice settings. *Research on Social Work Practice, 25*(4), 423–432. https://doi.org/10.1177/ 1049731514535989

Matamonasa-Bennett, A. (2015). "A disease of the outside people": Native American men's perceptions of intimate partner violence. *Psychology of Women Quarterly, 39*(1), 20–36. https://doi.org/10.1177/0361684314543783

Mathers, R. (2012). the failure of state-led economic development on American Indian reservations. *The Independent Review, 17*(1), 65–80. https://www.independent.org/pdf/tir/ tir_17_01_05_mathers.pdf

Okamoto, S. K., Kulis, S., Marsiglia, F. F., Steiker, L. K. H., & Dustman, P. (2013). A continuum of approaches toward developing culturally focused prevention interventions: From adaptation to grounding. *The Journal of Primary Prevention, 35*(2), 103–112. https://doi.org/10.1007/s10935-013-0334-z

Palinkas, L., Aarons, G., Chorpita, B., Hoagwood, K., Landsverk, J., & Weisz, J. (2009). Cultural exchange and the implementation of evidence-based practices: Two case studies. *Research on Social Work Practice, 19*(5), 602–612. https://doi.org/10.1177/ 1049731509335529

Pennington-Zoellner, K. J. (2009). Expanding community in the community response to intimate partner violence. *Journal of Family Violence, 24*(8), 539–545. https://doi.org/10.1007/s10896-009-9252-5

Smith, A. (2015). *Conquest: Sexual violence and American Indian genocide*. Duke Press.

Smith, C. A., Ireland, T. O., Park, A., Elwyn, L., & Thornberry, T. P. (2011). Intergenerational continuities and discontinuities in intimate partner violence: A two-generational prospective study. *Journal of Interpersonal Violence, 26*(18), 3720–3752. https://doi.org/10.1177/0886260511403751

Stewart, M., Makwarimba, E., Barnfather, A., Reutter, L., Letourneau, N., & Hungler, K. (2007). Promoting the health of vulnerable populations. *Diversity & Equality in Health and Care*. 33-48. https://diversityhealthcare.imedpub.com/promoting-the-health-of-vulnerable-populations-collaborative-research-strategies.pdf

Walters, K. L., & Simoni, J. M. (2009). Decolonizing strategies for mentoring American Indians and Alaska Natives in HIV and mental health research. *American Journal of Public Health, 99*(S1), S1. https://doi.org/10.2105/ajph.2008.136127

Whitaker, D. J., Baker, C. K., & Arias, I. (2008). Interventions to Prevent Intimate Partner Violence. In L. S. Doll, S. E. Bonzo, D. A. Sleet, & J. A. Mercy (Eds.), *Handbook of injury and violence prevention, 203-221*. Springer.

Yuan, N. P., Belcourt-Dittloff, A., Schultz, K., Packard, G., & Duran, B. M. (2015). Research agenda for violence against American Indian and Alaska Native women: Toward the development of strength-based and resilience interventions. *Psychology of Violence, 5*(4), 367. https://doi.org/10.1037/a0038507

Index

Note: Figures are indicated by *italics*. Tables are indicated by **bold**. Endnotes are indicated by the page number followed by 'n' and the endnote number e.g., 20n1 refers to endnote 1 on page 20.

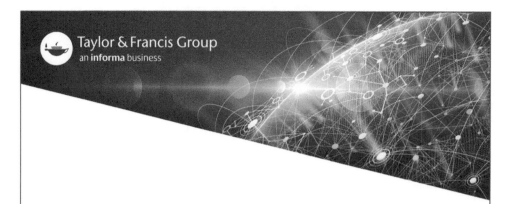

Taylor & Francis eBooks

www.taylorfrancis.com

A single destination for eBooks from Taylor & Francis
with increased functionality and an improved user
experience to meet the needs of our customers.

90,000+ eBooks of award-winning academic content in
Humanities, Social Science, Science, Technology, Engineering,
and Medical written by a global network of editors and authors.

TAYLOR & FRANCIS EBOOKS OFFERS:

A streamlined
experience for
our library
customers

A single point
of discovery
for all of our
eBook content

Improved
search and
discovery of
content at both
book and
chapter level

REQUEST A FREE TRIAL
support@taylorfrancis.com

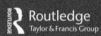 Routledge
Taylor & Francis Group

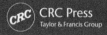 CRC Press
Taylor & Francis Group